Refractive Management of Ametropia

Refractive Management of Ametropia

Edited by

Kenneth E. Brookman, O.D., Ph.D., M.P.H.

Professor and Chairman
Department of Clinical Sciences
Southern California College of Optometry
Fullerton

Butterworth-Heinemann
Boston   Oxford   Melbourne   Singapore   Toronto   Munich   New Delhi   Tokyo

Copyright © 1996 by Butterworth-Heinemann

 A member of the Reed Elsevier group

Every effort has been made to ensure that the drug dosage schedules within this text are accurate and conform to standards accepted at time of publication. However, as treatment recommendations vary in the light of continuing research and clinical experience, the reader is advised to verify drug dosage schedules herein with information found on product information sheets. This is especially true in cases of new or infrequently used drugs.

Recognizing the importance of preserving what has been written, Butterworth-Heinemann prints its books on acid-free paper whenever possible.

Library of Congress Cataloging-in-Publication Data
Refractive management of ametropia / edited by Kenneth E. Brookman.
    p. cm.
  Includes bibliographical references and index.
  ISBN 0-7506-9569-2 (alk. paper)
    1. Eye—Refractive errors—Treatment. 2. Ophthalmic lenses.
  I. Brookman, Kenneth Edward, 1947–
    [DNLM: 1. Refractive Errors—therapy. WW 300 R333 1996]
  RE930.R44 1966
  617.7'55—dc20
  DNLM/DLC
  for Library of Congress   95-45065
                                                    CIP

British Library Cataloguing-in-Publication Data
A catalogue record for this book is available from the British Library.

The publisher offers discounts on bulk orders of this book.
For information, please write:
Manager of Special Sales
Butterworth-Heinemann
313 Washington Street
Newton, MA 02158-1626

10 9 8 7 6 5 4 3 2 1

Printed in the United States of America

Contents

Contributing Authors   *vii*
Preface   *ix*

1. Clinical Analysis and Management of Ametropia   1
        Kenneth E. Brookman

2. Myopia   13
        David A. Goss

3. Hyperopia   45
        Nancy B. Carlson

4. Astigmatism   73
        Robert C. Capone

5. Anisometropia   99
        Douglas K. Penisten

6. Low Ametropias   123
        Kenneth E. Brookman

7. Presbyopia   145
        Daniel Kurtz

Appendix: Answers to Clinical Questions   181

Chapter 2   181
Chapter 3   183
Chapter 4   186
Chapter 5   189
Chapter 6   192
Chapter 7   195

Glossary: List of Abbreviations and Symbols   *199*
Index   *201*

Contributing Authors

Kenneth E. Brookman, O.D., Ph.D., M.P.H.
*Professor and Chairman, Department of Clinical Sciences,
Southern California College of Optometry, Fullerton*

Robert C. Capone, O.D., F.A.A.O.
*Assistant Professor of Optometry, Department of External Clinics,
New England College of Optometry, Boston; Staff Optometrist, Eye
Services, East Boston Neighborhood Health Center, East Boston*

Nancy B. Carlson, O.D.
*Professor of Optometry and Chair, Department of Clinical
Skills and Practice, Chief of Staff, New England Eye Institute,
New England College of Optometry, Boston*

David A. Goss, O.D., Ph.D.
*Professor of Optometry, Indiana University School of Optometry,
Bloomington*

Daniel Kurtz, Ph.D., O.D.
*Professor of Optometry, Department of Clinical Skills and Practice,
New England College of Optometry, Boston*

Douglas K. Penisten, O.D., Ph.D.
*Associate Professor of Optometry, Northeastern State University
College of Optometry, Tahlequah, Oklahoma*

Preface

Management of ametropia has been the cornerstone of optometric practice since before its formal beginning nearly a century ago. *Refractive Management of Ametropia* is dedicated to this important aspect of practice because of its significance in eye and vision care and because optometrists provide this service to their patients more than any other.

The subject of prescribing spectacle lenses to manage ametropia is one that is difficult to teach and to learn because of the limited literature available addressing this topic and because there are different management philosophies for similar clinical problems. Some of these philosophies are anecdotal in nature ("clinical pearls"), which have been developed through personal clinical experience and observation. Others are based, at least in part, on scientific inquiry. In either case, optometry students, especially those who are beginning their patient care experience, must have an understanding of these approaches and the rationale for their use in order to develop their own clinical problem-solving and patient management skills.

This book was written as a teaching text for optometry students. However, practitioners of eye and vision care will find it a valuable resource as well. The organization of this book is designed to foster the readers' understanding of

- The subjective and objective patient problems resulting from the ametropias
- The factors that must be considered in the development of a refractive treatment plan
- The rationale for specific management approaches
- The clinical decision-making process

Each chapter of this book, excluding the first chapter, discusses the refractive management of a different type of ametropia. The first chapter provides an overview of clinical analysis and management of ametropia and includes a discussion of the general symptoms and signs of ametropia. Each of the subsequent chapters is divided into the following sections:

A CASE STUDY. This section includes an introductory case study of the subject ametropia. It is intended to "set the stage" for the subsequent discussion of symptoms and signs, clinical analysis, and refractive management.

SYMPTOMS AND SIGNS. This section addresses patient symptoms and clinical signs of the subject ametropia.

PRESCRIPTION CONSIDERATIONS AND GUIDELINES. This section discusses prescribing considerations and guidelines for the subject ametropia with respect to factors such as patient age, severity of the ametropia, patient lens wear history, effect of prescribing on accommodation and vergence, spectacle lens design, and vocational and avocational needs.

CASE STUDIES. This section includes a variety of clinical cases which present a patient history, clinical findings, assessment and treatment plan. Clinical findings omitted from a case presentation can be considered "normal" or "clinically insignificant" for the particular patient. The case studies are designed to illustrate different management strategies for the subject ametropia. Each case includes a discussion of the significant aspects of the case and the rationale for the recommended treatment plan.

SUMMARY. This section highlights key points discussed in the chapter to emphasize important issues related to the analysis and management of the subject ametropia.

CASE STUDY EXERCISES. Each chapter, excluding the first chapter, contains case study exercises to assist the reader in developing an understanding of the analysis and management of various types of ametropias. Sample solutions to these exercises are presented in the appendix.

The content of this book, like any discussion of clinical analysis and management, tends to be influenced to some degree by the personal philosophies and experiences of the authors. This helps to illustrate that there are a number of valid approaches to the same clinical problem. The authors of this book have discussed different approaches to specific clinical problems when appropriate.

Other publications are available that quite adequately address issues of the epidemiology, pathogenesis, pathophysiology, and clinical testing related to ametropia. These topics therefore are not emphasized. The focus of this book is refractive management with the clinical objectives of alleviating symptoms that result from ametropia and providing clear, comfortable, and efficient vision. The authors recognize that there are other management strategies that have clinical objectives of prevention and control of certain ametropias. These topics are addressed in other publications.

The readers of this book should keep in mind that because each patient presents a different set of circumstances and challenges, the management approach to what seem to be similar cases may vary. Other factors that may influence the disposition of an individual case are presented to justify the particular management strategy used.

Refractive Management of Ametropia would not have been possible without the expertise and clinical experience of a number of distinguished optometric faculty. I extend my sincere thanks and appreciation to Drs. Robert Capone, Nancy Carlson, David Goss, Daniel Kurtz, and Douglas Penisten for their dedicated effort and quality contribution to this work.

The advice and input from those other than the contributing authors of a book are also important to the quality of the manuscript. I therefore wish to thank John Griffin, O.D., M.S. for his assistance with the preparation of Chapter 1 and Ted Grosvenor, O.D., Ph.D. and John Ross for their assistance with the preparation of Chapter 2.

K. E. B.

1   Clinical Analysis and Management of Ametropia

Kenneth E. Brookman

Historical Notes

The art and science of refraction and prescribing spectacle lenses have formed the cornerstone of optometric practice since before the formal beginning of the profession during the late 19th and early 20th centuries. Although a specific time in history is difficult to identify as the origin of the profession per se, a knowledge of lenses and their application toward the enhancement of vision dates back many centuries.

Roger Bacon is often credited with the earliest use of ophthalmic lenses to correct refractive errors (presbyopia in particular) in the 13th century.[1,2] The notion of ametropia (refractive error) was mentioned much earlier by Aristotle but was ignored for many years that followed.

During the 20th century great strides have been made in refraction of the eye and management of ametropia with spectacle and contact lenses. Both objective and subjective refraction methods have improved during this century through the development of clinical techniques such as the Jackson crossed-cylinder, astigmatic dial, and binocular refraction (for example, vectograph) and through the development of instrumentation such as the retinoscope, phoropter, and automated refractor. New spectacle and contact lens designs and materials for the management of ametropia have contributed to the high quality of vision care provided by optometrists.

Symptoms and Signs of Ametropia

The causation of most anomalies of the eye and vision can be classified as refractive, integrative, organic, or psychogenic. Symptoms reported by patients can be very diagnostic in differentiating these causes. However, the differential diagnosis often can be difficult to make on the basis of patient symptoms alone, since many different anomalies may produce the same symptoms.[3] For any ametropia, refraction of the eye yields the primary diagnostic sign.

The two most commonly reported symptoms resulting from uncorrected or undercorrected ametropia are blurred vision and asthenopia, including asthenopic headache. Blurred vision is the most diagnostic symptom, since an ametropia usually causes some degree of decreased visual acuity.

Blurred vision is sometimes reported by patients as "double vision" with one eye or both eyes. This symptom, when resulting from ametropia, is not diplopia resulting from a loss of fusion, but rather is ghost imagery resulting from an out-of-focus image. This symptom is often due to uncorrected astigmatism. The differential diagnosis will likely be made between true diplopia due to a loss of fusion and ghost imagery if the symptom is eliminated with the best refractive correction.

The viewing distance at which blurred vision occurs and the degree of blur depends primarily on the type and severity of the ametropia, respectively, but also may be influenced by the age of the person and the level of illumination in the environment. Blurred vision may also be manifested and reported as a difficulty or inability to refocus between different viewing distances (that is, from far to near or from near to far).

Asthenopia is a term applied to a collection of related but often different symptoms. The *Dictionary of Visual Science* defines asthenopia as, "A term generally used to designate any subjective symptoms or distress arising from use of the eyes; eyestrain."[4] Asthenopia includes symptoms of headache, eye fatigue, pain around or above the eyes, photophobia, and eyestrain.[3] Eye pain that is sharp or burning is often associated with stress on the accommodation system, whereas pain that is pulling or drawing is often associated with stress on the convergence system. Uncorrected ametropia per se does not usually result in eye pain unless it adversely affects the accommodation or vergence system.

The causes of asthenopia are varied. Amos suggests that asthenopia results from "stress-related" tasks in association with " . . . uncorrected or undercorrected ametropia, muscle imbalance, improperly adjusted glasses, incorrect posture, or neurosis."[5] Each of these potential causes of asthenopia could be easily evaluated. Because small and moderate uncorrected ametropias are often the cause of symptoms of asthenopia, they should be considered the most probable diagnosis until clinical findings suggest otherwise.[3]

Headaches associated with asthenopia are often caused by uncorrected or undercorrected ametropia. Other causes are accommodation dysfunction and deficiencies of binocular vision skills, perhaps due to extended contraction of the ciliary or recti muscles.[6] Although the pathophysiology of this type of headache is unclear, there usually is a strong association between extended use of the eyes during a concentrated or stress-related vision task and the onset of a headache. This type of headache is usually an aching type pain of mild to moderate severity located in the temporal region of the head or at the canthi.[6] A patient history that establishes a relation between a headache and extended visual activity can be very diagnostic in terms of determining a cause and effect, especially if the headache resolves when the activity ceases or if the headache does not develop when the activity is avoided.

Chief complaints of blurred vision, asthenopia, or headache reported during a patient history require specific follow-up questioning to establish a diagnostic relation between the symptoms and specific vision tasks. This questioning should include the following areas with respect to the onset of symptoms:

- Viewing distance: far, near, or intermediate
- Time of day: morning, afternoon, or evening
- Type of visual activity: reading, video display terminal use, viewing a chalkboard in school, etc.
- Duration of the visual activity: immediately, after 15 minutes, after 60 minutes, etc.

The particular viewing distance at which the symptoms are noted may be significant in establishing the type of ametropia present. For example, blurred vision at far but not at near is most likely a result of myopia, whereas blur at near but not at far in a young patient would more likely be due to hyperopia. The time of day the symptoms occur and the type and duration of the visual activity are directed toward determining if the symptoms result from stress or fatigue. The severity of the condition is often indicated by the duration of the activity before the symptoms occur. The shorter the duration, the more severe the condition causing the symptoms is likely to be.

Any one or all of these symptoms might be manifested in a particular case. The intensity and frequency of the symptoms vary depending on a number of factors, including the severity of the ametropia, the type of ametropia, the integrity of the binocular vision system, the status of ocular health, and the nature of the vision tasks that cause the symptoms.

Uncorrected Ametropia and Visual Acuity

The relation between uncorrected ametropia and the resulting visual acuity has been investigated with respect to the type of ametropia and patient age.[7–10] Some investigators have proposed formulas that can be used to predict visual acuity from the amount of ametropia and vice versa.[9,10]

Eggers studied this relation among military personnel.[7] Table 1.1 summarizes Eggers' results. The data show that standard Snellen visual acuity decreases by approximately one line for each 0.25 diopter of uncorrected simple myopia or absolute (uncompensated) hyperopia. They also show that uncorrected astigmatism decreases visual acuity as a function of its magnitude and the axis of the correcting cylinder lens. For example, uncorrected oblique astigmatism (that is, the correcting cylinder axis is between either 31° and 59° or 121° and 149°) has a greater effect on visual acuity than either with-the-rule astigmatism (that is, the correcting cylinder axis is between either 150° and 180° or 180° and 30°), or against-the-rule astigmatism (that is, the correcting cylinder axis is between 60° and 120°). In other words, a greater amount of uncorrected with-the-rule or against-the-rule astigmatism will decrease visual acuity to the same degree as a lesser amount of oblique astigmatism.

Peters[8] and Hirsch[9] reported data similar to those of Eggers, although Hirsch found an average decrease in visual acuity from myopia to be slightly greater than one line per 0.25 diopter. Peters reported that although uncorrected distance visual acuity due to myopia remained constant with age, uncorrected visual acuity due to hyperopia decreased with age. For example, his data showed that for an age group of 5 to 15 years, 20/20 visual acuity was achieved with an uncorrected hyperopia as high as 2 diopters, whereas for an age group of 45 to 55 years, 20/20 acuity was achieved with hyperopia only as high as 1 diopter. A commonly accepted explanation for this decrease in acuity is that it is due to the reduction of the amplitude of accommodation that occurs with age, that is, the accommodation system is less able to clear a blurred image of a distant object resulting from uncorrected hyperopia.

A clinical rule-of-thumb with respect to the relation between uncorrected ametropia and visual acuity has resulted from these and other studies as well as from clinical observation. This rule-of-thumb may be stated as the following: *Snellen visual acuity decreases by one letter size on a standard test chart for every 0.25 diopter of uncorrected ametropia.* For example, if a best corrected visual acuity is considered to be 20/20, then a person with a 0.25 diopter of uncorrected simple ametropia, that is, myopia or absolute hyperopia, is expected to exhibit an uncorrected visual acuity of 20/25, or one line of acuity

TABLE 1.1   Visual Acuity as a Function of Uncorrected Ametropia

| Uncorrected Snellen Visual Acuity | Magnitude of Uncorrected Ametropia (D) | | |
| | Simple Myopia or Absolute Hyperopia | Simple Astigmatism* | |
		Oblique	With-the-Rule
20/25	0.25	—	0.50
20/30	0.50	0.75	1.00
20/40	0.75	1.00	1.50
20/50	1.00	1.50	2.00
20/70	1.25	1.75	2.50
20/100	1.50	2.25	3.00
20/150	2.00	2.75	3.50
20/200	2.50	3.50	4.50
20/250	3.00	4.25	5.50
20/300	3.50	5.00	6.25
20/350	4.00	—	—
20/400	4.50	—	—

*The values for against-the-rule astigmatism are considered to be about midway between oblique and with-the-rule.

(Adapted from Eggers 1945)

worse than 20/20. It follows that a 0.50 diopter of ametropia will result in an uncorrected acuity of 20/30, or two lines worse than 20/20, and so on.

Uncorrected astigmatism alone or in combination with myopia or hyperopia will also decrease visual acuity. However, to predict uncorrected visual acuity resulting from astigmatism, the concept of the *equivalent diopter sphere* (EDS) or *spherical equivalent* needs to be applied. The EDS represents an equivalent spherical ametropia when an emmetropia, simple myopia, or simple hyperopia is combined with astigmatism. The dioptric magnitude of the EDS is determined by adding one-half the magnitude of astigmatism to either emmetropia or the magnitude of the simple ametropia. For this calculation, the magnitudes of myopia and astigmatism are considered positive (+) values (that is, positive ametropias), hyperopia is considered a negative (–) value (that is, negative ametropia), and emmetropia is considered zero or plano. The refractive correction for these ametropias are of the opposite sign. That is, the correction for myopia and astigmatism is a negative (–) lens power and that for hyperopia is a positive (+) lens power.

The following three examples illustrate the application of the *equivalent diopter sphere* in predicting uncorrected visual acuity. Note that the EDS can also be predicted from an uncorrected visual acuity by use of the same concept.

1. The EDS of an eye with a simple myopia of 0.50 diopter (+0.50 D) combined with an against-the-rule astigmatism of 1.00 diopter (+1.00 D) equals *+0.50 D + (+1.00 D ÷ 2)*, or *1.00 D*. That is, the effect of the combination of the myopia and astigmatism would be the same as if the eye had only a simple myopia of 1.00 diopter. Using the rule of thumb, the predicted uncorrected visual acuity should be about 20/50 (that is, four acuity lines worse than 20/20). In this case, because both principal meridians of the eye are myopic, the ametropia is referred to as *compound myopic astigmatism.* The refractive correction for this eye would be *–0.50 –1.00 × 90.* The against-the-rule astigmatism suggests a correcting cylinder axis of 90°.

2. The EDS of an eye with a simple uncompensated hyperopia of 0.50 diopter (–0.50 D) combined with 1.00 diopter of with-the-rule astigmatism (+1.00 D) equals *–0.50 D + (+1.00 D ÷ 2)*, or plano, indicating that uncorrected visual acuity would be the same as if the eye were emmetropic. The predicted uncorrected visual acuity should be about 20/20. However, this eye would most likely have poorer uncorrected visual acuity than an emmetropic eye, because light from an distant object would not form a point focus at the retina as in emmetropia but would form a blurred circle because of the astigmatism. The result would be less than optimal acuity. In this case, because the horizontal principal meridian of the eye is hyperopic and the vertical is myopic, the ametropia is referred to as *mixed astigmatism.* The refractive correction for this eye would be *+0.50 –1.00 × 180.* The with-the-rule astigmatism suggests a correcting cylinder axis of 180°.

3. The EDS of an eye with emmetropia (plano) combined with 1.00 diopter (+1.00 D) of with-the-rule astigmatism equals *plano + (+1.00 D ÷ 2)*, or *0.50 D* of myopia (+0.50 D). The predicted uncorrected visual acuity would then be about 20/30. In this case, because the horizontal principal meridian of the eye is emmetropic and the vertical is myopic, the ametropia is referred to as *simple myopic astigmatism.* The refractive correction for this eye would be *plano –1.00 × 180.* The with-the-rule astigmatism suggests a correcting cylinder axis of 180°.

Rules-of-thumb, like those just described, are designed only as guidelines and are not absolutes. Thus caution must be exercised in application of the rules because there are exceptions. For example, the author's clinical experience suggests that Snellen visual acuity decreases by about one line of letters for every 0.25 to 0.50 diopter of simple ametropia, the average being 0.37 diopter per line for low to moderate ametropias. This value seems to be somewhere between that reported by Eggers[7] and Hirsch[9].

An understanding of the effect of uncorrected ametropia on visual acuity is important to the clinician because it provides a means to develop a preliminary diagnosis based on the patient history and habitual visual acuities. It also provides a means to confirm the internal consistency of clinical data between the symptoms a patient describes, visual acuity, and refraction data.

Suppose a patient presents with an uncorrected visual acuity of 20/60 measured at a distance of 6 meters. A refraction shows a correction of –0.50 DS (indicating 0.50 diopter of simple myopia) with a best corrected visual acuity of 20/20. If one then asks if the uncorrected visual acuity is consistent with the type and magnitude of the ametropia, the answer would have to be "no," because the acuity is worse than expected for the magnitude of the myopia (see Table 1.1). Therefore, either the patient truly has better uncorrected acuity than that measured or the ametropia is undercorrected. Considering this inconsistency, the clinician might then remeasure the acuity and refraction to confirm or refute the initial findings.

Fundamentals of Clinical Analysis

Clinical analysis is the process of relating a patient's symptoms to clinical signs toward the formulation of a diagnosis and treatment plan. In many ways, clinical analysis is similar to the method of scientific inquiry, what is commonly known as the *scientific method.* Table 1.2 illustrates the similarities of these two processes by comparing the steps of each.

The scientific method is usually initiated with a research question or problem for which a prediction (hypothesis) is proposed about the outcome of the inquiry. Similarly, clinical analysis is initiated by a prediction (preliminary or pre-diagnosis) of the most likely cause of symptoms and signs presented by a patient.[11] In the formulation of this prediction, the clinician considers a number of factors, including the relation among symptoms, clinical signs, and diagnoses, and the epidemiology of eye and vision conditions in the patient population. The clinician then conducts appropriate clinical tests and procedures to determine if the pre-diagnosis is confirmed. If this diagnosis is not confirmed after analysis of the clinical findings, additional tests and procedures may be indicated toward the formulation of an alternative diagnosis. The scientific investigator does essentially the same by conducting appropriate tests and measurements to either support or refute the hypothesis. Unlike clinical analysis, the scientific method may not require an alternative hypothesis and additional testing if the hypothesis is not confirmed. A scientific inquiry that supports a null hypothesis may be considered just as successful as one that does not. In either case, valid conclusions can be drawn from the results.

TABLE 1.2 Comparison of Clinical Analysis and the Scientific Method

Scientific Method	Clinical Analysis
Formulate a hypothesis from a scientific problem or question.	Formulate a preliminary diagnosis from symptoms and signs.
Design an experiment to obtain appropriate scientific data.	Perform appropriate clinical testing to obtain problem-related data.
Analyze the data to support or refute the hypothesis.	Analyze the clinical data to confirm the preliminary diagnosis.
Formulate conclusions from the results of the inquiry.	Design a treatment plan if the preliminary diagnosis is confirmed, or repeat the process if it is not.

When a diagnosis has been confirmed, the clinician develops a treatment plan, which may include treatment options, referral for further testing or consultation, patient education, and follow-up care. During clinical decision-making, clinicians often consider a series of questions that address important issues that relate to symptoms and signs, management considerations for the patient, and prognosis of the case. These questions that contribute to clinical decision-making are useful in providing a framework and rationale for the assessment and treatment strategy in each case. The following are examples of these clinical questions:

- Does the patient's chief complaint correlate with a specific uncorrected or undercorrected ametropia?
- Does information from the patient history other than the chief complaint provide clues to the severity and type of the ametropia?
- Does a comparison of the corrected and uncorrected visual acuities at distance and/or near correlate with the patient's symptoms, and objective and subjective refraction data?
- Are the measurements of refraction, that is, keratometry, retinoscopy, and subjective refraction, consistent with each other? What indicators suggest that they are not?
- Would prescribing spectacle lenses for a first-time lens wearer or changing a spectacle prescription for a habitual wearer likely eliminate the patient's chief complaint? Will the patient appreciate the benefit of the prescription? How should the benefits be demonstrated to the patient?
- Are symptoms from adaptation to a first-time prescription or to a change of a habitual prescription expected? If so, what might these symptoms be, and how should the patient be instructed with regard to this adaptation? Should the prescription be modified to minimize these symptoms; if so, how should the prescription be modified?

- Could prescribing spectacle lenses for a first-time lens wearer or changing a spectacle prescription for a habitual wearer create new symptoms resulting from the effect on accommodation or vergence? Should the prescription be modified to minimize these symptoms; if so, how should it be modified?
- If the patient uses spectacle lenses, do the lenses have design features, for example, base curve, thickness, segment height, that should be duplicated to minimize adaptation to a prescription change? If the lenses are for a first-time wearer, what design features, if any, would facilitate adaptation? Is the lens design compatible with the patient's vocational and avocational needs? If the lens design is not compatible, what modifications should be made?

Although there may be other clinically relevant questions that could be considered in an individual case, the ones presented herein are useful for general application.

Management of Ametropia with Spectacle Lenses

In most cases, the diagnosis of ametropia is relatively easy to make because the condition is the most common anomaly of the eye and vision and therefore is likely to be the cause of most symptoms. In addition, the correlation between a patient's symptoms and clinical signs (for example, visual acuity and refraction) is usually quite high. However, the presence of ametropia alone does not always provide justification for management with spectacle or contact lenses; each patient's needs must be considered and evaluated on an individual basis.

Indications or justifications for managing ametropia with spectacles or contact lenses include the following:[3,12,13]

- Improvement of visual acuity
- Restoration of comfortable vision by eliminating symptoms of asthenopia
- Enhancement of vision efficiency
- Prevention or slowing of the progression of ametropia
- Prevention of the development of secondary anomalies
- Protection and safety
- Special vocational or avocational requirements
- Cosmesis
- Mechanical support (for example, a ptosis crutch)

The management of ametropia may not be as straightforward as the diagnosis. Factors other than the correction of ametropia with spectacle or contact lenses must be considered for each patient before a prescription is written. These factors, many of which are mentioned earlier, include the patient's age, history of spectacle lens wear, vocational and avocational vision requirements, ability to adapt to change, type and severity of the ametropia, and the potential effect of the prescription on accommodation and vergence.

Milder and Rubin[14] present four practical principles of patient care that are applicable to the management of ametropia as well as to many other conditions. These principles are:

- Get the facts (historical and clinical).
- Use rules-of-thumb cautiously.
- *Primum non nocere,* or do no harm.
- Don't rock the boat.

The first principle suggests that before a treatment plan is developed and implemented, all pertinent information regarding the patient (that is, the patient history and clinical findings) must be obtained and evaluated. The second principle means that rules-of-thumb are designed as guidelines, not absolutes. Caution must be exercised in their application because the same rules are not appropriate for all situations.

The essence of the third principle is that the goal of any management strategy is to establish normal function and thereby eliminate symptoms and signs that result from a dysfunction or deficit. However, the creation of another dysfunction or deficit by achieving this goal must be avoided if at all possible.

The fourth principle certainly has widespread application. Patients can often be quite tolerant of less than perfect vision. For example, a patient may present completely satisfied with his or her visual acuity and comfort, although some changes have occurred. The principle suggests that for this patient, no change is recommended, to avoid creation of a problem when one did not exist. That is, change for the sake of change is not usually in the best interest of the patient.

References

1. Gregg JR. *The Story of Optometry.* New York: Ronald Press, 1965:47.
2. Hofstetter HW. *Optometry: Professional, Economic, and Legal Aspects.* St. Louis: Mosby, 1948:22.
3. Borish IM. *Clinical Refraction.* 2nd ed. Chicago: Professional Press, 1970:307–309;327–328.
4. Cline D, Hofstetter HW, Griffin JR. *Dictionary of Visual Science.* 4th ed. Radnor, Pa: Chilton, 1989:52.

5. Amos JF. Patient history. In: Eskridge JB, Amos JF, Bartlett JD, eds. *Clinical Procedures in Optometry.* Philadelphia: Lippincott, 1991:3–16.

6. Stelmack TR. Headache. In: Amos JF, ed. *Diagnosis and Management in Vision Care.* Boston: Butterworth-Heinemann, 1987:33–34.

7. Eggers H. Estimation of uncorrected visual acuity in malingerers. *Arch Ophthalmol* 1945;33:23–27.

8. Peters HB. The relationship between refractive error and visual acuity at three age levels. *Am J Optom Arch Am Acad Optom* 1961;38:194–198.

9. Hirsch MJ. Relation of visual acuity to myopia. *Arch Ophthalmol* 1945;34:418–421.

10. Singh K, Jain IS. Visual acuity in myopia. *Ind J Optom* 1967;1:6–13.

11. Eskridge JB. Decision making in patient care. In Eskridge JB, Amos JF, Bartlett JD, eds. *Clinical Procedures in Optometry.* Philadelphia: Lippincott, 1991:777–779.

12. Michaels DD. *Visual Optics and Refraction: A Clinical Approach.* 3rd ed. St. Louis: Mosby, 1985:457–483.

13. Michaels DD. Indications for prescribing spectacles. *Surv Ophthalmol* 1981;26:55–74.

14. Milder B, Rubin ML. *The Fine Art of Prescribing Spectacles Without Making a Spectacle of Yourself.* 2nd ed. Gainesville, Fla: Triad, 1991:3–4.

2 Myopia

David A. Goss

A Case Study of Myopia

History: R.S., an 11-year-old boy, was brought to the clinic by his parents because he said that he could not read the blackboard from the back of the classroom as his classmates could. He had never undergone an eye and vision examination. R.S. was doing well in school and liked to read, play baseball, and collect baseball cards. He was in good health.

Clinical Findings		6 m	40 cm
Habitual Visual			
Acuity (VA):	OD	20/60	20/20
	OS	20/60	20/20
Cover Test:		ortho	3$^\Delta$XP′
Near Point of Convergence (NPC): 3 cm			
Retinoscopy:	OD	$-1.00 -0.25 \times 180$	
	OS	-1.00 DS	
Subjective Refrac-			
tion (SRx):	OD	-1.00 DS (20/20)	
	OS	-1.00 DS (20/20)	

Phorometry (w/SRx):	6 m	40 cm
Phoria	ortho	2$^\Delta$EP′
Base-in (BI) Vergence	X/7/4	12/20/10
Base-out (BO) Vergence	12/18/8	24/32/14

Negative Relative Accom-
modation (NRA)/Positive
Relative Accommodation (PRA)   +2.25/–0.75
Amplitude of Accommodation (w/SRx): 14.25 D
Ocular Health, Tonometry, and Visual Fields: Normal OU

Assessment
1. Simple myopia OU
2. Higher than expected minimum amplitude of accommodation based on Hofstetter's age-related formulas.[1,2]
3. Esophoria at near with fusional vergence ranges that were within the normal ranges described by Morgan.[3,4]
4. Low positive relative accommodation.

Treatment Plan
1. Rx: OD   –1.00 DS
            OS   –1.00 DS
2. Lens design: Polycarbonate single vision lenses
3. Patient education: The prescription was for distance viewing only. R.S was advised that he could remove his spectacles for near work if he desired, but that he should remove them when reading for extended periods of time. This advice was appropriate because R.S. showed an esophoria at near while wearing the prescription, his PRA add was low, the amount of his myopia was small, and no astigmatism or anisometropia was present.

At a progress check one month after he received his glasses, R.S. reported that he could see much more in the distance and that his baseball hitting had improved. He was advised to return in 1 year for another complete eye and vision examination. It may be noted that at the initial examination the PRA was lower than might be predicted from the fact that the base-in fusional vergence ranges were normal.

Discussion
A low PRA in uncorrected myopia is a common finding. The PRA often increases after the prescription of lenses. In R.S.'s case, the PRA was –1.50 D at the progress check. Once myopia appears in childhood, it increases in amount. It is likely that R.S. will be found to have more myopia at next year's examination.

Symptoms and Signs of Myopia

The primary symptom of myopia is distance blur. As was patient R.S., children are often unaware of difficulty in distance viewing until they compare what they can see with what one of their friends or class-

TABLE 2.1   Amount of Myopia (Without Astigmatism) Typically Found with the Given Unaided Distance Visual Acuity Levels

Visual Acuity	Average Myopia (D)	95% Confidence Limit (D)
20/30	0.62	0.37–1.12
20/40	0.75	0.50–1.37
20/50	0.87	0.50–1.50
20/60	1.00	0.62–1.75
20/80	1.25	0.75–2.00
20/100	1.50	0.87–2.37
20/150	1.87	1.12–3.00
20/200	2.25	1.37–3.75
20/300	3.00	1.75–5.00
20/400	3.50	2.00–6.00
20/500	4.00	2.37–7.00
20/600	4.50	2.75–7.75
20/700	5.00	3.00–8.50
20/800	5.50	3.25–9.37
20/900	6.00	3.50–10.00
20/1000	6.50	3.75–10.62
20/1500	8.50	5.00–13.75
20/2000	10.25	6.00–16.50

(Modified from Hirsch MJ. Relation of visual acuity to myopia. *Arch Ophthalmol* 1945; 34:418–21. Copyright 1945 American Medical Association.)

mates sees. It is important to differentiate constant distance blur from intermittent distance blur. Intermittent distance blur is often a symptom of accommodative infacility. Asthenopia is usually not a problem in myopia unless the myopia is accompanied by astigmatism, anisometropia, accommodative dysfunction, or a vergence disorder. Symptoms of astigmatism may include distance and near blur or asthenopia.

The primary sign of myopia is reduced distance visual acuity. There is a close correlation between unaided distance visual acuity and amount of myopia. A chart with data from Hirsch (Table 2.1) can be helpful in seeing if the amount of myopia measured on the refraction is consistent with the unaided distance visual acuity.[5] Unaided near visual acuity is normal in myopia unless the amount is high enough that the nearpoint test distance is beyond the patient's far point of clear vision.

Classification and Prevalence of Myopia

Systems have been proposed over the years for the classification of myopia. Most of these systems have been flawed in some way because they have made assumptions about the cause of myopia or have required measurements (such as axial length) not always taken in the clinical setting. A useful way of classifying myopia is the system proposed by Grosvenor.[6] In this system myopia is classified by age of onset. The categories are congenital, youth onset, early adult onset, and late adult onset.

Congenital myopia is myopia present at birth that persists through infancy and childhood. It is often high in amount. The prevalence of congenital myopia is low, about 1% to 2%. Youth onset myopia is the most common form. The onset is from about 5 years of age to the teenage years or physical maturity. Once youth-onset myopia appears, the amount of myopia increases, a phenomenon sometimes referred to as myopia progression. The prevalence of myopia increases from about 2% at 6 years of age to about 20% at 15 years of age.[6–8] Early adult-onset myopia is myopia with onset in adulthood up to 40 years of age. The prevalence of myopia is 25% to 30% at 40 years of age. Myopia that appears after the age of 40 years is late adult-onset myopia. It seems to be less common than youth-onset and early adult-onset myopia.

Besides age, other factors affect myopia prevalence. One of these is ethnicity; the highest prevalences are among the Japanese and Chinese.[8–11] The prevalence of myopia increases with increases in family income.[7,8,12] The prevalence is greater among persons who have more years of education, and among persons who spend more time doing near work in their vocation and/or avocation.[7–16] Greater progression of myopia has been reported to be related to greater amount of time spent on close work and to closer working distance.[17] These associations of myopia with more near work have led many to assume that near work plays a role in the development of myopia.

Refractive Changes with Age

A wide range of refractive errors can be present at birth. Small amounts of myopia at birth usually disappear in the first year or two of life.[18,19] The presence of myopia in infancy may be a risk factor for the reappearance of myopia in the school years.[20] Children who enter school with spherical equivalent refractive conditions between emmetropia and 0.49 diopter of hyperopia are likely to become myopic by early teen age.[21]

The largest change in refractive error generally seen by the clinician in otherwise normal, healthy eyes is the increase in myopia seen among children after the youth onset of myopia.[22] These increases in myopia are usually referred to as *myopia progression.* In most young adults, refractive error is relatively stable, although the onset of and increases in myopia are not uncommon.

After the age of 45 years, there is a shift toward hyperopia. Between the ages of 45 and 70 years, the average shift toward more hyperopia or less myopia is between 0.75 and 1.00 diopter.[23] Shifts in the myopic direction in the sixth decade or later can also be associated with the development of age-related cataracts.

Progression of Myopia

Once myopia appears in childhood, it increases in amount, the myopia progression usually stopping or slowing in the middle to late teens.[24] Rates of childhood myopia progression in different studies are usually about 0.35 to 0.55 diopter per year, with standard deviations of about 0.25.[25–30] The earlier in childhood the onset of myopia, the faster is the rate of progression and the greater is the amount of myopia that has developed by the end of childhood.[30–33] The ocular optical component associated with childhood myopia progression is an increase in the depth of the vitreous chamber.[34–36]

Although childhood myopia progression typically stops or slows in the middle to late teens, further myopia progression can occur in adulthood. Mean rates of myopia increase in young adulthood reported in various studies usually are in the range of 0.02 to 0.10 diopter per year. Rates of up to 0.20 diopter per year sometimes are found among selected populations, such as persons in academic settings.[37–41]

Prescription Considerations and Guidelines

Although different patients have unique problems and challenges and patient care always requires carefully applied professional judgment, some general guidelines can be identified for the care of patients with myopia. Usually it is not necessary to correct myopia of less than 2.00 to 3.00 diopters in infants and toddlers. Myopia of this amount in infancy may disappear by about 2 years of age.[19] Also, the world with which infants interact is mostly close to them. It is appropriate to correct myopia of more than 1.00 to 1.50 diopters in preschool children, because the objects and persons with which and with whom they interact are farther away than in infancy. If myopia is not corrected at this time, it is advisable to examine the child at 6-month intervals.

As a child progresses through school, demands on distance vision and on near vision increase. Therefore, the minimum amount of myopia that is routinely corrected decreases with age while attention is paid to proper management of near vision problems. For children in the first few years of school, it may not be necessary to correct myopia less than 1.00 diopter. If the myopia is not corrected, it may be advisable to notify the child's teacher that the child is nearsighted. Because an increase in the myopia is expected, the child should be examined at 6-month intervals.

Most clinicians prescribe lenses to correct any amount of myopia in adolescents and adults whenever distance visual acuity is improved. Individuals differ in how critical they are about their distance visual acuity. Some persons report considerable improvement in acuity with correction of as little as 0.25 diopter of myopia. For these patients, prescriptions as small as –0.25 D can be written. For persons who are not sensitive to small dioptric steps, low prescriptions are not warranted.

For patients who are already wearing spectacles for myopia, a change of refractive error of 0.50 diopter from that in the patient's habitual prescription indicates that the prescription should be changed. Here also the patient's sensitivity to lens changes is important. Persons who are more critical about the clarity of their vision want a change in prescription when increases in myopia of as little as 0.25 diopter have occurred. A useful subjective procedure to help in deciding whether to make a small change in prescription is trial framing. With the patient viewing objects at distance, the patient is asked if clarity is noticeably improved with the addition of minus spheres over the habitual prescription in a trial frame or over the current glasses.

Uncorrected astigmatism can be responsible for asthenopia or reduced distance and near visual acuity. Because of this, cylinder lens corrections for 0.50 diopter or more should be routinely included in prescriptions for myopia (compound myopic astigmatism). It may not be necessary to include 0.25 diopter cylinders except when the patient notices considerable improvement with it or when a 0.25 diopter cylinder was included in a previously successful prescription. Uncorrected against-the-rule or oblique astigmatism is more often associated with symptoms than equal amounts of with-the-rule astigmatism. In simple myopic astigmatism, the decision to prescribe for astigmatism of 0.50 or 0.75 diopter depends on how critical is the patient about clear vision and how great are patient's visual demands. Correction of against-the-rule or oblique astigmatism is more likely than correction of with-the-rule astigmatism.

Because power varies with meridian in a cylindrical or spherocylindrical lens, magnification also varies with meridian. This causes some patients difficulty in adapting to the lenses. This is more likely when the amount of astigmatism is high and in oblique astigmatism. Children usually adapt without difficulty, although some children have problems initially with corrections for oblique astigmatism. When cylinders are prescribed for adults, patients should be warned that it will take some time to adapt to the lenses and that this adaptation will be more likely if they wear the lenses full time. Minus cylinder lenses and minimal vertex distance minimize meridional magnification and ease adaptation. If adaptation has not occurred after full-time wear for 2 weeks, reduction of the cylinder power may be necessary. If the cylinder power is reduced, the spherical power of the lenses must be adjusted to maintain the same spherical equivalent power.

Patients with myopia who are entering presbyopia often find that they can read without their glasses. This may be satisfactory if the patient has a low amount of myopia, does not have clinically significant amounts of astigmatism or anisometropia, and does not mind the inconvenience of removing the glasses for reading. This practice should not be encouraged for patients with high myopia. In this case the range of clear vision at near is likely to be closer than the patient's usual or convenient near working distance. This patient should be taught about the ranges of clear vision, and bifocal or progressive addition lenses should be recommended. It is not wise to delay the use of bifocal or progressive addition lenses because adaptation to them is easier when the addition powers are lower.

Accommodation and Vergence

In prescribing lenses for myopia it is important to consider characteristics of the patient's accommodation and convergence systems. For young patients with high exophoria and normal accommodative function, full-time wear of full minus correction may be recommended. Overcorrection of myopia is a treatment sometimes used for patients with exotropia.[42] Overcorrection of myopia stimulates accommodative convergence and reduces the amount of the exo deviation. In cases of esophoria at near, such as in convergence excess, and in cases of accommodative insufficiency, a nearpoint plus lens addition is recommended. The usual way that a near plus add is achieved is with bifocal or progressive addition lenses. Determination of the power of the plus add is covered in the literature on accommodation and convergence analysis.[42–46]

In esophoria at near, a useful way of determining the power of the plus add is to use just enough plus to make the near phoria ortho or low exo. One can make this determination by calculating the amount of plus lens addition necessary from the gradient accommodative convergence/accommodation (AC/A) ratio or by performing near phoria tests through different amounts of plus until the add that eliminates the esophoria is found. Plus adds also are used when there is an accommodative insufficiency. Another option in addition to bifocals and progressive addition lenses is that patients remove their glasses for nearpoint work if the amount of myopia is low and there is little or no astigmatism or anisometropia, as in patient R.S., whose case is discussed at the beginning of this chapter. A plus add for near may also be appropriate if exophoria at near is secondary to poor accommodative performance, that is, pseudo convergence insufficiency.[47,48]

Accommodation and convergence requirements are different with spectacle lenses and contact lenses.[49,50] More accommodation is required with minus contact lenses than with minus spectacle lenses. The difference in required accommodation increases as the amount of myopia increases. Patients with a moderate or high amount of myopia and borderline accommodative problems or approaching presbyopia may have nearpoint difficulties with contact lenses but not with spectacle lenses.

In dim illumination during distance viewing, a small amount of accommodation may be occurring rather than being at zero level. This is known as the *dark focus of accommodation* and is responsible for the phenomenon known as *night myopia*.[50–54] Some patients with low amounts of myopia or low amounts of simple myopic astigmatism may report blurred distance vision at night (often stated as when driving at night), but not at any other time. Correction of low myopia or low simple myopic astigmatism for nighttime seeing may be appropriate. For myopic patients already wearing spectacles and reporting distance blur at night, a potential technique for prescribing separate spectacles for night seeing is to perform retinoscopy under conditions in which room illumination has been turned off.[50,52–54]

Some patients with emmetropia or low amounts of hyperopia have overactive accommodation or difficulty in relaxing accommodation, often referred to as *accommodative excess* or *accommodative spasm*. This can result in apparent myopia or pseudomyopia.[50,55] Pseudomyopia most often occurs in young adults who are doing a great deal of near work. The diagnosis of pseudomyopia is confirmed when the manifest refraction is minus and a cycloplegic refraction is plano or plus. The presence of some or all of the following suggests a diagnosis of pseudomyopia and indicates that a cycloplegic refraction should be performed.

1. Asthenopia that is more severe than test findings suggest
2. Intermittent distance blur
3. Reduced and variable distance visual acuity
4. Low amplitude of accommodation for the patient's age
5. Low PRA or high negative relative accommodation (NRA) or both
6. Fluctuations in retinoscopic findings, subjective refraction, or pupil reflexes
7. More minus on subjective refraction than on static retinoscopy

Minus lenses should not be prescribed for pseudomyopia. The goal of treatment is to relax accommodation and eliminate the pseudomyopia. This is achieved with the prescription of any plus in the cycloplegic refraction for distance, plus lens additions for near work, and vision therapy designed to relax accommodation and improve fusional vergence ranges.[56–58] It is essential that the patient be taught about pseudomyopia, including the fact that distance vision may be blurred until accommodation is finally relaxed.

Measurement of Myopia

Many patients with myopia are very critical about clarity of vision. They may mistake increased darkness of letters at subjective refraction for improved visibility of letters. If the clinician is not careful about finding the proper end point at subjective refraction for these patients, the prescription will be too much minus. When minus is increased at the subjective refraction, the spherical end point has been passed if (a) the patient says that the previous lens was better, (b) the change does not allow the patient to read any more letters on the chart, or (c) the patient says the change makes the letters smaller and darker.

Many clinicians who perform examinations in 4-meter examination rooms record the subjective refraction measured in that room and then routinely add –0.25 D to the subjective refraction for the final prescription. This practice is used because the 4-meter test distance represents a 0.25 diopter accommodative stimulus rather than the zero accommodative stimulus that exists for optical infinity. It may also be noted that a 6-meter test distance, which is often assumed to represent optical infinity, actually has an accommodative stimulus of 0.167 diopter. A useful subjective procedure is to place lenses equal in power to the subjective refraction in a trial frame and show the patient the difference between that power and an additional –0.25 D as the patient looks at a distant object. The addition of the –0.25 D is confirmed if the patient notices a definite improvement.

Distance visual acuities with habitual correction can be useful in confirming refractive error changes from previous examinations. In the absence of amblyopia or reduction in visual acuity due to structural or pathologic cause, the eye that has the worse visual acuity with previous correction should also be the eye with the greatest increase in myopia.

Spectacle Lens Design

Correction for myopia can be provided in the form of spectacle lenses or contact lenses. Contact lenses are often the preferred form of correction for sports activities. Many patients also prefer contact lenses for cosmetic reasons. Patients with high amounts of myopia sometimes subjectively report better vision with contact lenses, perhaps because there is less image minification with minus contact lenses than with minus spectacle lenses.

Lens reflections can be bothersome to users of low minus spectacle lenses. These reflections can be reduced with an antireflection coating on both surfaces of the lenses. For higher minus power lenses, the weight of the lenses and the appearance of the greater edge thickness in minus lenses become important considerations.[59–61] Antireflection coatings also can be beneficial by improving the appearance of the lens. The size and shape of the spectacle frame influence the appearance of the lenses. To minimize edge thickness, smaller eye sizes and high index materials should be used. A rounded lens results in thinner edges overall than would exist in some parts of a square or rectangular lens. A thick eyewire on the spectacle frame conceals the edge better than a thin eyewire or rimless design.

Special edging procedures help conceal the thick edges of lenses. First, hide-a-bevel lens construction, in which the bevel is placed further forward on the lens, allows the front surface of the lens to be flush with the front of the spectacle frame. Second, one can order a procedure known as rolling and polishing, in which the edge thickness is reduced before the lens is inserted in the frame. It is advisable to use an antireflection coating with rolling and polishing, because the latter procedure can cause reflections to be conspicuous at the lens edge. The use of aspheric lenses is also helpful in reducing weight and edge thickness.

Another potential cosmetic problem with high minus spectacle lenses is the appearance of rings caused by reflections from the lens edges. The appearance of these rings can be minimized by coating the edge of the lens, buffing the edge, using hide-a-bevel construction, or using an antireflection coating.

Weight of spectacle lenses can be minimized by use of lenses with lower densities and higher refractive index values. CR-39 is a very widely used hard resin material for spectacle lenses. However, polycarbonate lenses are lighter because polycarbonate has a higher refractive index and a lower density than CR-39 resin. The refractive index of 1.586 for polycarbonate can be compared to 1.498 for CR-39 resin, 1.523 for crown glass, and 1.56 to 1.66 for polyurethane. Refractive index is a factor in weight and thickness of lenses because a higher refractive index means a less bulky lens. High-index materials have a higher percentage of incident light reflected from them, so concomitant use of an antireflection coating is advisable. Polycarbonate lenses are the lenses of choice for safety considerations and sports activities because they have the greatest impact resistance of any currently available lens material.

High minus lenses are sometimes made with relatively flat front surface base curves. Lenses with base curves flatter than about +2.50 D have a poor appearance because there is considerable reflection from the front surface of the lenses.

Accuracy of the lens prescription is important in high minus corrections. The interpupillary distance must be accurately determined, because errors induce unwanted prismatic effects. Vertex distance is another important consideration. Vertex distance is the distance from the back surface vertex of the correcting lens to the apex of the cornea. For a given myopic eye, the minus power necessary to correct the eye decreases as vertex distance decreases. The following effective power formula can be used to calculate the power of the correcting lens when vertex distance is changed:

$$F_2 = \frac{F_1}{1 - dF_1}$$

where F_1 = power in diopters of the correcting lens at the initial location
         F_2 = power in diopters needed in a correcting lens placed at a second location

d = distance in meters from the plane of the initial correcting lens to the plane of the second correcting lens, the sign being negative if the second lens is farther from the eye than the initial lens and positive if the second lens is closer to the eye than the initial lens

Vertex distance can be measured with an instrument called a *distometer.* One can also determine vertex distance by placing a ruler lightly against the patient's closed eyelid and recording the distance to the spectacle lens plane in the trial frame or spectacle frame. This procedure also can be performed with a phoropter if the phoropter is one in which the lens wells are empty at the zero power setting. About 1 millimeter should then be added for eyelid thickness. For patients with a high amount of myopia, spectacle plane vertex distance should be specified when refractions are performed and when lenses are ordered. If there is a change in vertex distance (as for instance, from one pair of spectacles to another or from a spectacle plane refraction to the corneal plane for contact lens wear), the new power should be calculated with the formula. Another alternative is to find the subjective end point with a trial frame with the lenses at the appropriate vertex distance.

With contact lenses, it is important to perform careful overrefractions with the contact lenses in place. Vertex distance is especially important in contact lenses fitting. If the contact lens power needed (F_2) is calculated from a spectacle plane refractive error (F_1) of –4.50 D at a vertex distance of 14 mm (d = 0.014 meter), F_2 is equal to –4.23 D. Thus, a patient who needs a –4.50 D spectacle lens requires a power of only –4.25 D in a contact lens. The difference increases as the refractive correction increases.

Control of Myopia

Prescription of lenses when the primary consideration is the provision of clear distance vision for patients with myopia can be called *myopia correction.* Some clinicians design treatment regimens to try to slow myopia progression. This is often referred to as *myopia control.* Many clinicians recommend undercorrection or part-time wear as possible ways of slowing myopia progression. There are not enough published data on these methods to evaluate their efficacy in slowing myopia progression.

A common method of myopia control is bifocal lenses. Studies of the effect of bifocal lenses on the rate of childhood myopia progression have had mixed results.[62] In some studies, the investigators did not find a statistically significant effect of bifocals.[33,63,64] Other investigators reported reduced rates of progression with bifocals.[65–69] Differences in study outcomes are probably due to differences in method. Additional research has indicated myopia control with bifocals depends on particular test findings.[66,67,70–72] In one study, investigators

TABLE 2.2   Mean Rates of Increase in Childhood Myopia as a Function of Near-point Phoria and Spectacle Lens Type

Study	Single Vision Lenses			Bifocal Lenses		
	n	Mean	SD	n	Mean	SD
Roberts and Banford						
Ortho and exo	181	0.41	—	17	0.38	—
Eso	167	0.48	—	65	0.28	—
Goss						
>6 exo	9	0.47	0.31	3	0.48	0.22
Ortho to 6 exo	27	0.43	0.21	18	0.45	0.27
Eso	10	0.54	0.30	35	0.32	0.20
Goss and Grosvenor						
>6 exo	5	0.50	0.26	6	0.43	0.23
Ortho to 6 exo	20	0.43	0.32	41	0.42	0.27
Eso	7	0.51	0.22	18	0.31	0.31

Note.—Data are from three studies.[66,67,70,71] Dash indicates data not reported.

found lower rates of progression with bifocals in children with higher intraocular pressures.[72]

Three studies showed a reduction in the rate of childhood myopia progression of about 0.2 diopter per year with bifocals in patients with nearpoint esophoria.[66,67,70,71] The results of these studies are summarized in Table 2.2. Because a plus lens addition for near is indicated in nearpoint esophoria, a bifocal can be recommended in these cases for reasons in addition to potential myopia control. In recommending a bifocal to the patient and parents, it is helpful to first demonstrate that the lens power through which the patient sees most clearly at distance is not the same as the lens power through which the patient sees most clearly and comfortably at near. This is usually the case in nearpoint esophoria. It can then be explained that the way these different powers are incorporated into a lens is by the use of a bifocal. If the word *bifocal* is mentioned before this demonstration, sometimes parents remark that they thought bifocals were for older people. The data in Figure 2.1 show that rates of childhood myopia progression are lowest when the habitual nearpoint phoria is orthophoria or low exophoria. This suggests that the best add power for myopia control would be just enough plus to make the near phoria ortho or low exo. This is also a common way of prescribing nearpoint plus adds for relief of asthenopia.[46] Progressive addition lenses also have been used for patients without presbyopia,[73,74] but the effectiveness of these lenses for myopia control has not been studied.

Rigid gas-permeable contact lenses can be used for myopia control. In a 3-year study, 56 children who wore rigid gas-permeable contact lenses had a mean rate of myopia increase of 0.16 diopter per year, compared with a mean rate of increase of 0.51 diopter per year for a

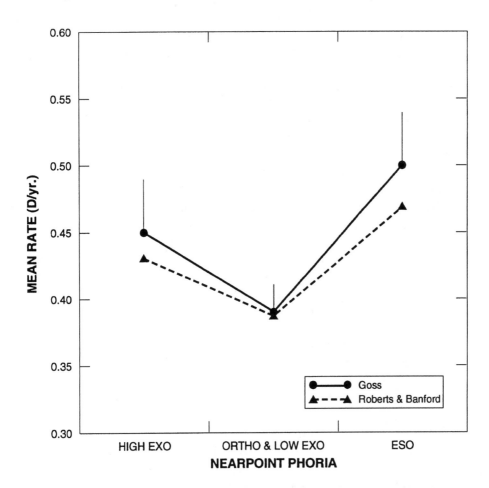

FIGURE 2.1   *Mean rates of childhood myopia increase in diopters per year as a function of habitual nearpoint phoria from two studies. Data from the study by Roberts and Banford[66,67] are for wearers of single-vision lenses. Data from the study by Goss[30] include both wearers of single-vision lenses and wearers of bifocal lenses. The habitual phoria for bifocal wearers was calculated from the AC/A ratio. The ortho and low exo grouping was from orthophoria to 4 prism diopters exophoria in the study by Roberts and Banford and from orthophoria to 6 prism diopters exophoria in the study by Goss. The error bars indicate one standard error.* (Reprinted with permission from Goss DA. Effect of spectacle correction on the progression of myopia in children. *J Am Optom Assoc* 1994:65:117–128.)

control group who wore spectacle lenses.[75] The investigators attributed the difference to corneal flattening induced by the contact lenses.[75,76] The change in corneal power as measured with keratometry over the 3 years varied from no change to a flattening of 1.25 diopters with a mean change of 0.37 diopter flattening. Thus part of the difference between the contact lens wearers and the spectacle lens wearers could be accounted for by corneal changes as assessed with keratometry. The rest of the difference was probably due to changes at the corneal apex, which is not measured with keratometry.[75,76] Twenty-three of the subjects in the study agreed to not wear their contact lenses for 2.5 months after the completion of the study. The mean changes in myopia for these 23 subjects were an increase of 0.76 diopter during 44 months of contact lens wear followed by an increase of 0.27 diopter during the 2.5 months when contact lenses were not worn.[76] Mean changes in corneal power as measured with keratometry for these 23 subjects were a decrease of 0.27 diopter during the 44 months of contact lens wear and an increase of 0.25 diopter during the 2.5 months when the contact lenses were not worn. Therefore, it appears that rigid gas-permeable contact lenses can be used to control myopia progression by means of corneal flattening, but there can be a rebound effect if contact lens wear is discontinued.

Some optometrists recommend vision therapy to improve accommodation and convergence function and provide suggestions for visual hygiene for myopia control.[77–79] These visual hygiene suggestions include guidelines for patients such as those that follow:

1. Take a break from reading or near work about every 30 minutes. During this break stand up, walk around the room, and look out the window.
2. Use a relaxed upright posture while reading. Sit in a comfortable chair with a straight back.
3. Use adequate illumination for reading. Avoid glare on the page by using a diffuse light source directed over your shoulder from behind you.
4. To check for a proper working distance while you are reading, make a fist and hold it up against your nose. Your book should be at least as far away as your elbow.
5. Sit at least 6 feet away when watching television.
6. Limit the time each day you spend watching television and playing video games.
7. Get some physical exercise each day.

There is no direct evidence that such behaviors aid in myopia control, but they appear to be good recommendations irrespective of possible myopia control effects.

Case Studies of Myopia

Patient M.P.

History: M.P., a 9-year-old girl, complained of distance blur with her habitual (current) spectacle lenses (HRx). Her last eye and vision examination was about 1 year before the current visit. Her parents mentioned that she did well in school and that she read extensively.

M.P., in fact, brought a book with her to the examination to read in the waiting room.

Clinical Findings		6 m	40 cm
Habitual VA:	OD	20/30	20/20 with −2.25 −0.25 × 80
	OS	20/40⁻¹	20/20 with −2.00 −0.25 × 95
Cover test (w/HRx):		ortho	ortho'
NPC: 2 cm			
Retinoscopy:	OD	−3.00 −0.25 × 90	
	OS	−3.00 −0.25 × 90	
Subjective Refraction (SRx):	OD	−3.00 −0.25 × 75 (20/15)	
	OS	−3.00 −0.25 × 105 (20/15)	

Phorometry (w/SRx):	6 m	40 cm
Phoria	ortho	5ᐃEP'
BI vergence	X/8/3	6/18/4
BO vergence	10/20/10	24/32/15
NRA/PRA		+2.25/−1.00
Gradient AC/A ratio		6/1

Amplitude of Accommodation (w/SRx): 15.00 D

Ocular Health, Tonometry, and Visual Fields: Normal OU

Trial Frame: M.P. was instructed to look at distance and compare her vision with her habitual lenses and with −0.75 D OD and −1.00 D OS held over her habitual lens. She said that things were clearer with the additional lenses. She was then asked to make the same comparison when looking at the print in her book. She stated that her eyes felt a little more comfortable and the letters were a little bigger without the additional lenses.

Assessment
1. Increase in myopia OU (OS > OD)
2. Convergence excess
3. Low base-in fusional range and low PRA at near

Treatment Plan
1. Rx: OD   −3.00 −0.25 × 75   +1.00 D add
       OS   −3.00 −0.25 × 105   +1.00 D add
   An add power of +1.00 D was chosen because the gradient AC/A ratio indicated that this add was the minimum necessary to shift the near phoria into the normal range of between orthophoria and 6 prism diopters exophoria.
2. Lens Design: Polycarbonate FT-35 mm bifocal lenses
3. Patient Education: M.P. and her parents were informed that the myopia had increased and that M.P. would need new glasses to

once again improve her distance vision. Her parents asked about when the increases in myopia would stop and whether there was anything that could be done to slow it. They were informed that the myopia would likely increase at least until M.P. reached physical maturity in her mid teens. They were also told that one way that myopia can sometimes be slowed, but not stopped, was to use different lens powers for distance and near.

Discussion
M.P. exhibited a little more increase in myopia in her left eye than in her right eye. This is consistent with the fact that her left eye distance visual acuity with correction was a little worse than with her right eye. Because M.P. had esophoria at near through the subjective refraction, she may have slowing of her myopia progression with a bifocal lens.[70,71] The binocular vision case type in which M.P. would be categorized is convergence excess.[44,46,80] A plus add is the treatment of choice for convergence excess.

Patient A.G.

History: A.G., a 28-year-old junior high school teacher, reported for an eye and vision examination because he noticed a slight blur at distance with his current glasses. He enjoyed yard work, and during the summer he worked on a house construction crew. His history was otherwise unremarkable.

Clinical Findings		4 m	40 cm
Habitual VA:	OD	20/20	20/20 with −1.25 −0.50 × 175
	OS	20/20	20/20 with −1.50 −0.25 × 180
Cover Test (w/HRx):		ortho	ortho'
Retinoscopy:	OD	−1.75 −0.25 × 180	
	OS	−1.50 −0.50 × 180	
SRx:	OD	−1.50 −0.50 × 180 (20/20^{+2})	
	OS	−1.50 −0.50 × 180 (20/20^{+1}) OU (20/15^{-2})	

Phorometry (w/SRx):	4 m	40 cm
Phoria	1$^\Delta$XP	4$^\Delta$XP'
BI vergence	X/9/4	14/22/10
BO vergence	12/22/7	17/28/9
NRA/PRA		+2.25/−2.25

Ocular Health, Tonometry, and Visual Fields: Normal OU

Assessment
1. Slight increase in myopia OS and slight increase in astigmatism OD

2. Phorias, vergence ranges, and NRA/PRA within normal ranges defined by Morgan

Treatment Plan
1. Rx: OD $-1.75 -0.50 \times 180$
        OS $-1.75 -0.50 \times 180$
2. Lens Design: Polycarbonate single vision lenses
3. Patient Education: A.G. was told that he had noticed blurred distance vision because he had an increase in his "nearsightedness." He was also told that the new prescription would restore clear distance vision.

Discussion
The differences in the spherical equivalents from the habitual prescription to the patient's refraction were -0.25 D OD and -0.12 D OS. There was a 5° change in right eye cylinder axis, which generally is not clinically significant for a 0.50 diopter cylinder. These changes would usually not be large enough to warrant a change in prescription. The examination was conducted in a 4-meter examination room. When -0.25 D is added to the refraction to compensate for the test distance, the difference from the habitual prescription becomes OD -0.50 D, OS -0.37 D. This is usually enough change to be noticeable to the patient. When lenses equal in power to the difference from the habitual prescription were held over the habitual prescription, the patient observed an improvement in clarity for distance.

Patient L.M.

History: L.M., a 40-year-old elementary school teacher, reported for an annual eye and vision examination expressing an interest in contact lenses. L.M.'s vocational and avocational vision requirements included reading, computers, and tennis. She was not having any problem with her current glasses. Her history was otherwise unremarkable.

Clinical Findings		6 m	40 cm
Habitual VA:	OD	20/15	$20/20^{-2}$ with -6.00 DS
	OS	20/15	$20/20^{-2}$ with -8.00 DS
Cover Test (w/SRx):		ortho	8^{Δ}XP'
NPC: 4 cm			
Retinoscopy:	OD	$-6.00 -0.50 \times 90$	
	OS	$-8.25 -0.25 \times 90$	
SRx:	OD	$-6.00 -0.25 \times 95$ (20/15)	
	OS	$-8.00 -0.25 \times 75$ (20/15)	

Phorometry (w/SRx):	6 m	40 cm
Phoria	2ΔXP	7ΔXP'
BI vergence	X/8/4	16/24/18
BO vergence	12/24/15	X/32/14
NRA/PRA		+2.25/–1.00

Ocular Health, Tonometry, and Visual Fields: Normal OU

Assessment

1. No change of myopia but the presence of a 0.25 diopter astigmatism OU
2. Near dissociated phoria (7ΔXP') was outside the normal range defined by Morgan, but the near base-out range was more than twice the amount of the phoria, and the patient had no symptoms.
3. No contraindications to contact lens wear

Treatment Plan

1. No change of the current spectacle prescription.
2. L.M. scheduled a soft contact lens fitting.
3. Patient Education: L.M. was informed that no change in the current spectacle prescription was needed. She was told that she might have difficulty with near work while wearing contact lenses, because of the increased demand on accommodation and the positioning of the contact lenses with near viewing. She indicated that she would still like to try them. Soft contact lenses were fitted successfully.

Discussion

The low PRA can be attributed to approaching presbyopia. More accommodation is required with minus contact lenses than minus spectacle lenses, the difference increasing as the amount of myopia increases. Because of approaching presbyopia and her fairly high amount of myopia, L.M. might have had difficulty accommodating for near objects with contact lenses even though she did not have any problem with spectacle lenses.

At the 2-week contact lens progress check, L.M. confirmed that she was having difficulty reading with her contact lenses. The various correction options were explained to her. She decided to use progressive addition lenses with plano sphere in the distance portion of the lenses. She used the prescribed reading addition of +1.00 D for classroom work, and she used her spectacles when reading for extended periods of time at home. L.M. also wore her contact lenses for tennis. She obtained plano power sports protective goggles for tennis.

Patient G.W.

History: G.W., a 47-year-old business executive presented with main vision needs related to computer use and paperwork. He liked to go bicycling in his spare time. He reported having a slight blur at near. He did not notice any difficulty at distance. G.W.'s current spectacle prescription was 3 years old. His history was otherwise unremarkable.

Clinical Findings		6m	40 cm
Habitual VA:	OD	20/20	20/30 with −2.75 −2.50 × 173
	OS	20/20	20/30 with −2.25 −3.00 × 15
			+1.25 D add OU
Cover Test (w/HRx):		ortho	9$^\Delta$XP′
Retinoscopy:	OD	−2.25 −2.25 × 170	
	OS	−2.25 −2.50 × 10	
SRx:	OD	−2.25 −2.25 × 170 (20/15)	
	OS	−2.00 −2.50 × 15 (20/15)	

Tentative Add at 40 cm: +1.25 D (20/20)

Phorometry (w/SRx):	6 m	40 cm (w/+1.25 D add)
Phoria	2 XP	9$^\Delta$XP′
BI vergence	X/12/8	17/24/12
BO vergence	X/20/12	X/27/12
NRA/PRA		+1.25/−1.00
Fixation Disparity		Zero

Trial Frame: During a demonstration of the new distance and near prescription in a trial frame, G.W. stated that his near vision was very good with the new lens powers.

Ocular Health, Tonometry, and Visual Fields: Normal OU

Assessment
1. Decrease in myopia and decrease in with-the-rule astigmatism OU

Treatment Plan
1. Rx: OD −2.25 −2.25 × 170 +1.25 D add
      OS −2.00 −2.50 × 15   +1.25 D add
2. Lens Design: Polycarbonate progressive addition lenses
3. Patient Education: G.W. was informed that he had experienced a small change in the lens correction needed for clear vision at distance.

Discussion

The changes of ametropia exhibited by G.W. are expected after about 45 years of age. The spherical equivalent minus correction decreased by 0.62 diopter in the right eye and by 0.50 diopter in the left eye. The add power was the same as in his previous prescription, but his near vision was improved with the new correction because the total minus power for near was less because of the decreased minus in the distance correction. The new distance correction also gave a small improvement in distance visual acuity.

Patient M.R.

History: M.R. was a 33-year-old mail carrier with a walking route. She was not having any vision problems. It had been 2 years since she had undergone an eye and vision examination, and she wanted to get a new spectacle frame. Her history was otherwise unremarkable.

Clinical Findings		6 m	40 cm
Habitual VA:	OD	$20/20^{-2}$	20/20 with $-2.25 -0.25 \times 70$
	OS	$20/25^{+3}$	20/20 with $-2.00 -0.25 \times 105$
Cover Test (w/HRx):		4^{Δ}XP	9^{Δ}XP′
Amplitude of Accommodation (w/HRx): 8.00 D			
Retinoscopy:	OD	$-2.50 -0.25 \times 90$	
	OS	$-2.50 -0.50 \times 95$	
SRx:	OD	$-2.50 -0.50 \times 75$ $(20/15^{-2})$	
	OS	$-2.25 -0.50 \times 105$ $(20/15^{-1})$	

Phorometry (w/SRx):	6 m	40 cm
Phoria	4^{Δ}XP	7^{Δ}XP′
BI vergence	X/10/7	15/23/12
BO vergence	9/15/8	14/19/8
NRA/PRA		+1.50/−2.50
Gradient AC/A ratio		4/1

Assessment

1. Increase in myopia and astigmatism by 0.25 diopter each OU, that is, the spherical equivalent changed from the habitual prescription by −0.37 D in each eye
2. Low to moderate exophoria at distance and near with positive fusional vergence ranges (blur points), which just equal twice the phorias

Treatment Plan

1. Rx: OD $-2.50 -0.50 \times 75$
   OS $-2.25 -0.50 \times 105$

2. Lens Design: Polycarbonate single vision lenses
3. Patient Education: M.R. was informed that she had experienced a slight change in her distance prescription.

Discussion

The change in ametropia exhibited by M.R. might not be enough to make a change in prescription, especially if the patient is not experiencing distance blur. However, in M.R.'s case there were three reasons for deciding to change the prescription to that measured on the subjective refraction: (a) M.R. wanted to get a new spectacle frame. The prescription should be updated for the new glasses. (b) When −0.37 D spheres were held over M.R'.s habitual spectacle lenses she said that she did notice a small improvement in her distance vision. (c) M.R.'s phoria findings correspond to the basic exophoria binocular vision case type. Though M.R. had no symptoms, it is generally advisable to fully correct myopia in basic exophoria as long as accommodation findings are normal. If myopia is undercorrected, the exophoria is increased because less accommodative convergence occurs.

Patient B.C.

History: B.C. was a 61-year-old farm homemaker. She enjoyed nature walks and writing poetry about nature and farm life. She stated that she could not see fine print as well as when she got her glasses 2 years earlier. She reported no problems with her distance vision. B.C.'s general health was good, and she was taking no medication. The history was otherwise unremarkable.

Clinical Findings		6 m	40 cm
Habitual VA:	OD	20/20^{-2}	20/30^{-1} with −1.75 −1.25 × 163
	OS	20/20^{-2}	20/30^{-1} with −1.00 −1.25 × 179
			+2.00 D add OU
Cover Test (w/HRx):		ortho	7$^{\Delta}$XP′
Retinoscopy:	OD	−1.50 −1.00 × 180	
	OS	−1.00 −1.00 × 180	
SRx:	OD	−1.50 −1.00 × 178 (20/20^{-1})	
	OS	−0.75 −1.00 × 02 (20/20^{-1})	

Tentative Add at 40 cm: +2.25 D (20/20)

Phorometry (w/SRx):	6 m	40 cm (w/+2.25 D add)
Phoria	1$^{\Delta}$EP	8$^{\Delta}$XP′
Fixation disparity		Zero

Trial Frame: B.C. reported that her near vision was improved when she viewed through the new lens powers in a trial frame.
Ocular Health, Tonometry, and Visual Fields: Normal for age

Assessment

1. Slight decrease in myopia and with-the-rule astigmatism (that is, the spherical equivalents of the subjective refraction were 0.37 diopter less minus than the habitual lens powers) and a change in axis of the correcting cylinder OD

Treatment Plan

1. Rx: OD   −1.50 −1.00 × 180   +2.25 D add
          OS   −0.75 −1.00 × 02   +2.25 D add
2. Lens Design: CR-39 resin FT-25 bifocal lenses
3. Patient Education: B.C. was told that she had experienced a small change of her prescription at distance and near.

Discussion

The decrease in myopia correction and the 0.25 diopter increase in add power resulted in an increase of 0.62 diopter in the total near-point plus power. This improved B.C.'s near vision. The change in the distance prescription made only a one-letter acuity improvement in B.C.'s distance vision.

Summary

The fundamental goals in vision care for patients with myopia are the same as for any other patient, that is, to provide clear, comfortable, efficient vision at both distance and near. Clear vision for distance is achieved by prescribing minus lenses in powers determined with careful retinoscopic and subjective refraction procedures. For clear vision at near, it may be necessary to use a plus add if the patient also has an accommodation or convergence dysfunction or presbyopia. To make sure the patient has comfortable and efficient vision, it is important that the clinician carefully and comprehensively examine accommodation and convergence function and provide appropriate lens, prism, or vision therapy management.

Myopia can be classified as congenital, youth onset, early adult onset, and late adult onset. The most common is youth onset. Once myopia appears in childhood, it increases in amount. This is referred to as *myopia progression*. Childhood myopia progression typically slows or stops in the middle to late teens. Onset or additional progression of myopia also can occur in adulthood. The symptom associated with myopia is decreased distance visual acuity. The minimum amount of myopia that should be corrected decreases as visual demands at intermediate and far distances increase. Thus for adolescents and adults, myopia as little as 0.25 diopter can be corrected if it results in improved distance visual acuity. Similarly, changes in prescription of as little as 0.25 diopter can be made if the patient notices an appreciable improvement in acuity. More commonly, however, lenses are changed when there are refractive error changes of 0.50 diopter or more. If no modifications in the prescription are indicated by the accommodation and convergence findings, the lenses prescribed for persons with myopia are typically the binocular maximum plus (actually the minimum minus) subjective refraction that provides best visual acuity.

The symptoms of astigmatism include asthenopia and reduced distance and near visual acuity. For some patients, uncorrected astigmatism of as little as 0.50 diopter can cause vision problems. This is more likely in against-the-rule astigmatism than in with-the-rule astigmatism. Cylinder corrections for 0.50 diopter or more astigmatism should be included in prescriptions for compound myopic astigmatism. Adults who have not previously worn a correction for astigmatism or who have had a change in astigmatism should be told that they should expect some changes in their perception of shapes and distances until they adapt to the new lenses. They should be instructed to wear the new glasses full time for 2 weeks to allow this adaptation to occur. For patients who do not adapt to cylinder changes, the cylinder power can be reduced. If the cylinder power is reduced, it is important to maintain the spherical equivalent power in the correction.

When spectacle lenses are prescribed, an important consideration is the design features. The most careful and comprehensive examination and the most exact lens prescription can still be followed by patient dissatisfaction if the spectacles are fabricated incorrectly, are cosmetically unappealing, or are too heavy. These factors are especially important in high myopia.

Many clinicians are concerned about controlling myopia progression so that the amount of myopia developed is not as great as would otherwise occur. Some of the most common methods of attempted myopia control are bifocal lenses, rigid contact lenses, and proper visual hygiene. The literature suggests that bifocals can reduce the rate of childhood myopia progression in some patients—an average reduction of about 0.2 diopter per year in children with nearpoint esophoria. It appears that rigid gas-permeable contact lenses reduce the rate of childhood myopia progression by flattening the cornea.

References

1. Hofstetter HW. A useful age-amplitude formula. *Penn Optom* 1947;7:5–8.

2. Goss DA. *Ocular Accommodation, Convergence, and Fixation Disparity: A Manual of Clinical Analysis.* 2nd ed. Boston: Butterworth-Heinemann, 1995:120–121.

3. Morgan MW. Analysis of clinical data. *Am J Optom Arch Am Acad Optom* 1944;21:477–491.

4. Goss DA. *Ocular Accommodation, Convergence, and Fixation Disparity: A Manual of Clinical Analysis.* 2nd ed. Boston: Butterworth-Heinemann, 1995:62–64.

5. Hirsch MJ. Relation of visual acuity to myopia. *Arch Ophthalmol* 1945;34:418–421.

6. Grosvenor T. A review and a suggested classification system for myopia on the basis of age-related prevalence and age of onset. *Am J Optom Physiol Opt* 1987;64:545–554.

7. Sperduto RD, Seigel D, Roberts J, Rowland M. Prevalence of myopia in the United States. *Arch Ophthalmol* 1983;101:405–407.

8. Working Group on Myopia Prevalence and Progression. *Myopia: Prevalence and Progression.* Washington, DC: National Academy Press, 1989:8–22,45–61.

9. Borish IM. *Clinical Refraction.* 3rd ed. Chicago: Professional Press, 1970:19–28.

10. Baldwin WR. A review of statistical studies of relations between myopia and ethnic, behavioral, and physiological characteristics. *Am J Optom Physiol Opt* 1981;58:516–527.

11. Bear JC. Epidemiology and genetics of refractive anomalies. In: Grosvenor T, Flom MC, eds. *Refractive Anomalies: Research and Clinical Applications.* Boston: Butterworth-Heinemann, 1991:57–80.

12. Angle J, Wissman DA. The epidemiology of myopia. *Am J Epidemiol* 1980;111:220–228.

13. Goldschmidt E. *On the Etiology of Myopia: An Epidemiological Study.* Copenhagen: Munksgaard, 1968:25–59.

14. Peckham CS, Gardiner PA, Goldstein H. Acquired myopia in 11-year-old children. *Br Med J* 1977;1:542–544.

15. Angle J, Wissman DA. Age, reading, and myopia. *Am J Optom Physiol Opt* 1978;55:302–308.

16. Richler A, Bear JC. Refraction, nearwork and education: a population study in Newfoundland. *Acta Ophthalmol* 1980;58:468–478.

17. Parssinen O, Lyyra AL. Myopia and myopic progression among schoolchildren: a three-year follow-up study. *Invest Ophthalmol Vis Sci* 1993;34:2794–2802.

18. Ingram RM, Barr A. Changes in refraction between the ages of 1 and 3 1/2 years. *Br J Ophthalmol* 1979;63:339–342.

19. Mohindra I, Held R. Refraction in humans from birth to five years. *Doc Ophthalmol* 1981;28:19–27.

20. Gwiazda J, Thorn F, Bauer J, Held R. Emmetropization and the progression of manifest refraction in children followed from infancy to puberty. *Clin Vis Sci* 1993;8:337–344.

21. Hirsch MJ. Predictability of refraction at age 14 on the basis of testing at age 6: interim report from the Ojai longitudinal study of refraction. *Am J Optom Arch Am Acad Optom* 1963;40:127–132.

22. Hofstetter HW. Some interrelationships of age, refraction, and rate of refractive change. *Am J Optom Arch Am Acad Optom* 1954;31:161–169.

23. Hirsch MJ. Refractive changes with age. In Hirsch MJ, Wick RE, eds. *Vision of the Aging Patient.* Philadelphia: Chilton, 1960:63–82.

24. Goss DA, Winkler RL. Progression of myopia in youth: age of cessation. *Am J Optom Physiol Opt* 1983;60:651–658.

25. Nolan JA. Progress of myopia with contact lenses. *Contacto* 1964;8:25–26.

26. Baldwin WR, West D, Jolley J, Reid W. Effects of contact lenses on refractive, corneal, and axial length changes in young myopes. *Am J Optom Arch Am Acad Optom* 1969;46:903–911.

27. Rosenberg T, Goldschmidt E. The onset and progression of myopia in Danish school children. *Doc Ophthalmol* 1981;28:33–39.

28. Mantyjarvi MI. Changes of refraction in school children. *Arch Ophthalmol* 1985;103:790–792.

29. Goss DA, Cox VD. Trends in the change of clinical refractive error in myopes. *J Am Optom Assoc* 1985;56:608–613.

30. Goss DA. Variables related to the rate of childhood myopia progression. *Optom Vis Sci* 1990;67:631–636.

31. Septon RD. Myopia among optometry students. *Am J Optom Physiol Opt* 1984;61:745–751.

32. Mantyjarvi MI. Predicting of myopia progression in school children. *J Pediatr Ophthalmol Strab* 1985;22:71–75.

33. Grosvenor T, Perrigin DM, Perrigin J, Maslovitz B. Houston myopia control study: a randomized clinical trial. II. Final report by the patient care team. *Am J Optom Physiol Opt* 1987;64:482–498.

34. Tokoro T, Kabe S. Relation between changes in the ocular refraction and refractive components and development of the myopia. *Acta Soc Ophthalmol Jpn* 1964;68:1240–1253.

35. Fledelius HC. Ophthalmic changes from age of 10 to 18 years: a longitudinal study of sequels to low birth weight. IV. Ultrasound oculometry of vitreous and axial length. *Acta Ophthalmol* 1982;60:403–411.

36. Goss DA. Childhood myopia. In: Grosvenor T, Flom MC, eds. *Refractive Anomalies: Research and Clinical Applications.* Boston: Butterworth-Heinemann, 1991:81–103.

37. Shotwell AJ. Plus lenses, prisms, and bifocal effects on myopia progression in military students. *Am J Optom Physiol Opt* 1981;58:349–354.

38. Goss DA, Erickson P, Cox VD. Prevalence and pattern of adult myopia progression in a general optometric practice population. *Am J Optom Physiol Opt* 1985;62:470–477.

39. Zadnik K, Mutti DO. Refractive error changes in law students. *Am J Optom Physiol Opt* 1987;64:558–561.

40. Goss DA, Erickson P. Meridional corneal components of myopia progression in young adults and children. *Am J Optom Physiol Opt* 1987;64: 475–481.

41. Working Group on Myopia Prevalence and Progression. *Myopia: Prevalence and Progression.* Washington, DC: National Academy Press, 1989:23–35,62–88.

42. Rutstein RP, Marsh-Tootle W, London R. Changes in refractive error for exotropes treated with overminus lenses. *Optom Vis Sci* 1989;66:487–491.

43. Cooper J. Accommodative dysfunction. In: Amos JF, ed. *Diagnosis and Management in Vision Care.* Boston: Butterworth, 1987:431–454.

44. Wick BC. Horizontal deviations. In: Amos JF, ed. *Diagnosis and Management in Vision Care.* Boston: Butterworth, 1987:461–510.

45. Birnbaum MH. *Optometric Management of Nearpoint Vision Disorders.* Boston: Butterworth-Heinemann, 1993:161–168.

46. Goss DA. Determining the optimal nearpoint plus prescription based on case types and examination test results. *J Behav Optom,* in press.

47. Goss DA. *Ocular Accommodation, Convergence, and Fixation Disparity: A Manual of Clinical Analysis.* 2nd ed. Boston: Butterworth-Heinemann, 1995:34–36.

48. Richman JE, Cron MT. *Guide to Vision Therapy.* South Bend, Ind: Bernell, 1987:17–18.

49. Westheimer G. The visual world of the new contact lens wearer. *J Am Optom Assoc* 1962;34:135–138.

50. Goss DA, Eskridge JB. Myopia. In: Amos JF, ed. *Diagnosis and Management in Vision Care.* Boston: Butterworth, 1987:121–171.

51. Leibowitz HW, Owens DA. Night myopia and the intermediate dark focus of accommodation. *J Opt Soc Am* 1975;65:1121–1128.

52. Owens DA, Leibowitz HW. Night myopia: cause and a possible basis for amelioration. *Am J Optom Physiol Opt* 1976;53:709–717.

53. Owens DA, Mohindra I, Held R. The effectiveness of a retinoscope beam as an accommodative stimulus. *Invest Ophthalmol Vis Sci* 1980;19:942–949.

54. Owens RL, Higgins KE. Long-term stability of the dark focus of accommodation. *Am J Optom Physiol Opt* 1983;60:32–38.

55. Stenson SM, Raskind RH. Pseudomyopia: etiology, mechanisms and therapy. *J Pediatr Ophthalmol* 1970;7:110–115.

56. Pollack SL, Grisham JD. Orthoptics for pseudomyopia. *Rev Optom* 1980;117:35–38.

57. Apodaca DB. Vision therapy for pseudomyopia. *Optom Monthly* 1984;75:397–399.

58. Scheiman M, Wick B. *Clinical Management of Binocular Vision: Heterophoric, Accommodative, and Eye Movement Disorders.* Philadelphia: Lippincott, 1994:360–364.

59. Brooks CW, Borish IM. *System for Ophthalmic Dispensing*. Chicago: Professional Press, 1979:50–51.

60. Krefman R. A better way to handle high Rx patients. *Optom Management* 1994;29:39–41.

61. Fannin TE, Grosvenor T. *Clinical Optics*. Boston: Butterworth, 1987:382–388.

62. Goss DA. Effect of spectacle correction on the progression of myopia in children: a literature review. *J Am Optom Assoc* 1994;65:117–128.

63. Schwartz JT. Results of a monozygotic cotwin control study of a treatment for myopia. In: *Twin Research 3: Epidemiological and Clinical Studies*. New York: Liss, 1981:249–58.

64. Parssinen O, Hemminki E, Klemetti A. Effect of spectacle use and accommodation on myopia progression: final results of a three-year randomized clinical trial among schoolchildren. *Br J Ophthalmol* 1989;73:547–551.

65. Miles PW. A study of heterophoria and myopia in children some of whom wore bifocal lenses. *Am J Ophthalmol* 1962;54:111–114.

66. Roberts WL, Banford RD. Evaluation of bifocal correction technique in juvenile myopia. O.D. dissertation. Massachusetts College of Optometry, 1963:108–124.

67. Roberts WL, Banford RD. Evaluation of bifocal correction technique in juvenile myopia. *Optom Weekly* 1967;58:25–28,31;58(39):21–30;58(40):23–28;58(41):27–34;58(43):19–24,26.

68. Oakley KH, Young FA. Bifocal control of myopia. *Am J Optom Physiol Opt* 1975;52:758–764.

69. Neetens A, Evens P. The use of bifocal as an alternative in the management of low grade myopia. *Bull Soc Belge Ophthalmol* 1985;214:79–85.

70. Goss DA. Effect of bifocal lenses on the rate of childhood myopia progression. *Am J Optom Physiol Opt* 1986;63:135–141.

71. Goss DA, Grosvenor T. Rates of childhood myopia progression with bifocals as a function of nearpoint phoria: consistency of three studies. *Optom Vis Sci* 1990;67:637–640.

72. Jensen H. Myopia progression in young school children: a prospective study of myopia progression and the effect of a trial with bifocal lenses and beta blocker drops. *Acta Ophthalmol* (Suppl 200)1991;33–37.

73. Valentino JA. Clinical use of progressive addition lenses on nonpresbyopic patients. *Optom Monthly* 1982;73:513–515.

74. Smith JB. Progressive-addition lenses in the treatment of accommodative esotropia. *Am J Ophthalmol* 1985;99:56–62.

75. Perrigin J, Perrigin D, Quintero S, Grosvenor T. Silicone-acrylate contact lenses for myopia control: 3-year results. *Optom Vis Sci* 1990;67:764–769.

76. Grosvenor T, Perrigin D, Perrigin J, Quintero S. Rigid gas-permeable contact lens for myopia control: effects of discontinuation of lens wear. *Optom Vis Sci* 1991;68:385–389.

77. Nolan JA. An approach to myopia control. *Optom Weekly* 1974;65:149–154.

78. Birnbaum MH. Clinical management of myopia. *Am J Optom Physiol Opt* 1981;58:554–559.

79. Birnbaum MH. *Optometric Management of Nearpoint Vision Disorders.* Boston: Butterworth-Heinemann, 1993:303–309.

80. Grosvenor TP. *Primary Care Optometry* 2nd ed. New York: Professional Press, 1989:344.

Case Study Exercises

For each case study presented, determine the diagnosis and develop a treatment plan. The clinical questions provided with each case may assist you by highlighting important aspects of the case.

Patient J.B.

History: J.B., a 10-year-old girl, presents blurred vision at distance with her current prescription. She does well in school and likes to read and to play basketball.

Clinical Findings		6 m	40 cm
Habitual VA:	OD	$20/60^{-1}$	20/20 with $-1.75 -1.25 \times 95$
	OS	20/60	20/20 with $-2.00 -0.50 \times 80$
SRx:	OD	$-2.75 -1.00 \times 90$ (20/15)	
	OS	$-2.75 -0.75 \times 80$ (20/15)	

Phorometry (w/SRx):	6 m	40 cm
Phoria	1^{Δ}EP	6^{Δ}EP′
BI vergence	X/6/3	14/22/12
BO vergence	X/20/14	26/34/22
NRA/PRA		+2.25/–0.50
Gradient AC/A Ratio		6/1

Clinical Questions
1. Is the patient's chief complaint consistent with the test findings?
2. Are the distance visual acuities with the habitual prescription consistent with the change in refractive error?
3. What are the options for myopia control?
4. What is your plan for patient treatment?
5. What lens prescription would you use?

Patient K.C.

History: K.C. is a 32-year-old graduate student in history. He reports slight distance blur and ocular discomfort after reading for 30 to 60 minutes. As a student, K.C. does an extensive amount of reading. His spectacle prescription is about 2 years old.

Clinical Findings		6 m	40 cm
Habitual VA:	OD	$20/25^{+3}$	20/20 with $-5.00 -1.25 \times 177$
	OS	$20/25^{+2}$	20/20 with $-3.50 -1.50 \times 04$
SRx:	OD	$-5.25 -1.25 \times 180$ ($20/20^{-1}$)	
	OS	$-3.75 -1.75 \times 07$ (20/20)	

Phorometry (w/SRx):   **6 m**   **40 cm**

	6 m	40 cm
Phoria	2^ΔXP	5^ΔXP'
BI vergence	X/9/5	22/27/20
BO vergence	X/10/6	14/20/12

Accommodation Testing: Accommodative insufficiency
Dynamic Retinoscopy at 40 cm: +1.00 D add

Clinical Questions

1. Are the symptoms consistent with the test findings?
2. Is having the patient remove his glasses for near work a reasonable option? Why or why not?
3. What is your plan for patient management?
4. What lens prescription would you recommend?

Patient C.B

History: C.B., a 35-year-old manager of a fast-food restaurant, reports no vision problems with her current spectacle lenses. She feels it is time for a check-up. Her hobby is gardening. Her history is otherwise unremarkable.

Clinical Findings		**4 m**	**40 cm**
Habitual VA:	OD	$20/20^{-2}$	20/20 with −1.50 −0.50 × 180
	OS	$20/20^{-2}$	20/20 with −1.50 −0.25 × 170
SRx (at 4 m):	OD	−1.75 −0.25 × 180 $(20/20^{+1})$	
	OS	−1.50 −0.50 × 173 $(20/20^{+2})$	

Phorometry: All accommodation and convergence findings are within normal limits

Clinical Questions

1. Is the patient's reported lack of vision problems consistent with the test findings?
2. Taking the 4-meter test distance into account, what are the spherical equivalent changes in the right eye and left eye from the habitual prescription?
3. Would "trial framing" be useful for this patient? Why or why not?
4. Would you recommend to this patient that she needs new glasses? Why or why not? If so, what lens prescription would you use?

Patient F.E.

History: F.E., a 15-year-old boy, states he thinks he has had another increase in his nearsightedness. He is a good student, is on his school's basketball and track teams, plays baseball, and does some yard and farm work.

Clinical Findings		6 m	40 cm
Habitual VA:	OD	20/30	20/20 with −4.25 DS
	OS	20/30^{+1}	20/20 with −4.50 DS
SRx:	OD	−4.75 DS (20/20^{+2})	
	OS	−4.75 −0.50 × 180 (20/20^{+3})	

Phorometry: All accommodation and convergence findings are within normal limits

Clinical Questions
1. Is the chief complaint consistent with the test findings?
2. Would you consider recommending contact lenses? Why or why not?
3. If contact lenses are used, what adjustment is made for vertex distance?
4. What lens prescription would you recommend?

Patient A.H

History: A.H., a 43-year-old college professor, has difficulty reading with his current spectacle lenses. His distance vision with these lenses is fine. His hobbies are reading and hiking. His history is otherwise unremarkable.

Clinical Findings		6 m	40 cm
Habitual VA:	OD	20/20^{+2}	20/30 with −2.50 −0.50 × 175
	OS	20/20^{+3}	20/30 with −2.75 −0.25 × 10
SRx:	OD	−2.50 −0.50 × 170 (20/20^{+3})	
	OS	−2.75 −0.25 × 15 (20/20^{+3})	

Tentative Add at 40 cm: +1.00 D (20/20)
Phorometry at 40 cm with SRx and +1.00 D Add:
  Phoria: 7$^{\Delta}$XP′
  Fixation disparity: zero

Clinical Questions
1. In light of the patient's age, what does the patient's chief complaint indicate?
2. If the patient had not been having any vision difficulty at all, would you change his lens prescription on the basis of the change in the refractive correction?
3. What lens prescription would you recommend?

3 Hyperopia

Nancy B. Carlson

A Case Study of Hyperopia

History: P.C., a 35-year-old arborist, presented for a routine eye examination. He had worn glasses for near only since age 32 and had lost them 3 months before his examination. P.C. reported that his vision was good at distance but that he was uncomfortable reading or performing close work without his glasses. P.C.'s general health was good. He was taking no medications and had no allergies. The family history was unremarkable.

Clinical Findings		6 m	40 cm
Habitual Visual			
Acuity (VA):	OD	20/25	20/20
	OS	20/25	20/20
Cover Test:		ortho	ortho'
Stereo Acuity at 40 cm:	70 seconds (Randot)		
Retinoscopy:	OD	plano −0.75 × 180	
	OS	plano −0.75 × 180	
Subjective Refrac-			
tion (SRx):	OD	+1.00 −1.00 × 10 (20/15)	
	OS	+1.00 −0.75 × 165 (20/15)	
Phorometry (w/SRx):		**6 m**	**40 cm**
Phoria		1$^\Delta$XP	5$^\Delta$XP'

Negative Relative Accom-
   modation (NRA)/ Positive
   Relative Accommodation (PRA)   +2.50/–2.00

Trial Frame: The subjective finding was trial framed, and the patient reported clear, comfortable vision with the lenses at both distance and near.

Assessment
1. Simple hyperopic astigmatism (with-the-rule) OD and compound hyperopic astigmatism (with-the-rule) OS

Treatment Plan
1. Rx: OD   +1.00 –1.00 × 10
        OS   +1.00 –0.75 × 165
2. Lens Design: Crown glass single vision lenses with photochromatic tint as the patient requested for indoor and outdoor use
3. Patient Education: P.C. was instructed to wear the lenses for all near work and for distance as needed and to return for re-examination in 2 years. He was advised that he should put on his glasses as soon as he started reading or performing close work rather than waiting for his eyes to become tired before putting on his glasses. P.C. was also told that as he aged he could expect to be wearing his glasses for distance as well as for near.

P.C. was examined 2 years later at the age of 37 years. He reported that he had been wearing his glasses full time for the past year. He said that his vision was good at distance without correction but that because he had been doing more close work for the past year, he was wearing his glasses more frequently and found it a nuisance to keep taking them off and putting them on. He had noticed that his vision was as good at distance with the glasses as it was without them. He reported no problems and stated that his vision was clear and comfortable at both distance and near with his current prescription. Further history was unremarkable.

Clinical Findings During Re-examination

Habitual VA:		6 m	40 cm
	OD	20/15	20/20 with +1.00 –1.00 × 10
	OS	20/15	20/20 with +1.00 –0.75 × 165
Retinoscopy:	OD	+2.25 –1.00 × 10	
	OS	+1.75 –0.75 × 165	
SRx:	OD	+2.00 –1.00 × 10 (20/15)	
	OS	+1.75 –1.00 × 165 (20/15)	

The subjective refraction finding was trial framed, and the patient reported that his vision was clear and comfortable at distance and near with the increased plus prescription. The subjective refraction was prescribed for full-time wear to correct P.C.'s increased manifest hyperopia. P.C. was examined 2 years later at 39 years of age. He reported no problems with his current prescription.

Clinical Findings During Second Re-examination

Habitual VA:		6 m	40 cm
	OD	20/20	20/25 with +2.00 –1.00 × 10
	OS	20/15	20/20 with +1.75 –1.00 × 165
Retinoscopy:	OD	+2.75 –0.75 × 10	
	OS	+2.50 –0.75 × 165	
SRx:	OD	+2.50 –1.00 × 10 (20/15)	
	OS	+2.25 –1.00 × 165 (20/15)	

Because P.C. again showed an increase in manifest hyperopia, the subjective refraction finding was prescribed for full-time wear. P.C. presented again for examination at 43 years of age. He reported that his vision was clear at distance with his current prescription but that his vision was intermittently blurry at near and he became tired after reading for more than 20 minutes.

Clinical Findings During Third Re-examination

Habitual VA:		6 m	40 cm
	OD	20/15	20/30 with +2.50 –1.00 × 10
	OS	20/15	20/30 with +2.25 –1.00 × 165
Retinoscopy:	OD	+2.50 –1.00 × 10	
	OS	+2.25 –1.00 × 165	
SRx:	OD	+2.50 –1.00 × 10 (20/15)	
	OS	+2.25 –1.00 × 165 (20/15)	

Tentative Add at 40 cm: +1.00 D (20/20)
NRA/PRA (w/+1.00 D add): +0.75/–0.50
Range of Clear Vision (w/+1.00 D add): 25 cm to greater than arm's length

Treatment Plan
1. Rx: There was no change in P.C.'s refraction, but because he was showing signs and symptoms of presbyopia, an add was prescribed. The prescription was as follows:
   OD   +2.50 –1.00 × 10 +1.00 D add
   OS   +2.25 –1.00 × 16 +1.00 D add
2. Lens Design: Polycarbonate lenses and a progressive addition lens design

Discussion

P.C.'s chief complaint (that is, discomfort at near) at the initial examination (age 32) is typical of a young adult with hyperopia. Persons with uncorrected hyperopia have a higher accommodative demand at near than do persons with emmetropia because they must accommodate for the working distance and to neutralize the hyperopia.

For distance, vision will be clear without correction provided the amplitude of accommodation is sufficient to compensate for hyperopic error. P.C.'s initial prescription is unknown because he had lost it before his examination at age 35. His refraction at age 35 of 1 diopter of hyperopia with some with-the-rule astigmatism is consistent with his complaint of discomfort with near vision and with his uncorrected visual acuity of 20/25 at distance and 20/20 at near. The slight decrease in distance vision of 20/25 is more likely to be related to the with-the-rule astigmatism rather than to the hyperopic error.

P.C.'s expected amplitude of accommodation for his age is 5.50 diopters according to Donders' table,[1] which is sufficient to neutralize his hyperopic error and give him clear distance vision without correction. The 1 diopter of hyperopia, however, in addition to a 40 cm working distance demand of 2.50 diopters, necessitates the use of 3.50 diopters of accommodation for near. With an amplitude of accommodation of only 5.50 diopters and an accommodative demand of 3.50 diopters, the patient would be expected to have asthenopic symptoms, because patients are generally comfortable if they are using half or less of their available amplitude.

The static retinoscopy finding at P.C.'s first visit showed less plus than the subjective refraction rather than the typical finding in hyperopia of more plus on retinoscopy than manifest in a dry refraction. This is probably due to inappropriate fog used during retinoscopy. However, because the process of subjective refraction includes fogging, the maximum plus manifest refraction was determined. Persons with hyperopia sometimes can relax their accommodation as fog is slowly reduced during the subjective refraction but find that the prescription makes their distance vision blurry once their habitual accommodation comes into play. Lenses for persons with hyperopia should be carefully trial framed to be sure that they do not decrease the patient's visual acuity. Because P.C. had near symptoms only and would be wearing his new prescription for near only, the distance visual acuity through the lenses was of less importance than his comfort when using the glasses for near vision.

P.C.'s positive response to the trial framing of the lenses was an important part of the decision about the prescription. He reported that he was comfortable with the prescription for near and that his vision was good through the prescription for distance. He was told to wear the glasses for near work, because that was when he experienced discomfort. He was also told that he could use the glasses for distance as needed, because his vision improved from 20/25 to 20/15 with the prescription. It was expected that P.C. would have little need for a distance prescription in his outdoor job. However, when he returned 2 years later, P.C. had found it more convenient to wear his glasses full time, as persons with hyperopia frequently do.

Over the next several years as more of his hyperopia became manifest, P.C.'s prescription was increased accordingly. At each examination, the results of the subjective refraction were trial framed and P.C. was asked to look out the window to be sure that his distance vision was still clear. P.C. also was asked to read at near with the increased plus prescription to be sure he was comfortable.

Symptoms and Signs of Hyperopia

Hyperopia is a refractive error frequently encountered by optometrists. The decisions about what to prescribe or not to prescribe are complex. Visual acuity is frequently unaffected in hyperopia, but patients are often uncomfortable or exhibit functional problems if the hyperopia is not corrected. Because persons with hyperopia habitually accommodate and often have difficulty relaxing accommodation in response to plus lenses, the optometrist cannot simply perform a refraction and prescribe lenses. Factors that must be considered in prescribing lenses for persons with hyperopia include the patient's symptoms, occupation, visual needs, age, degree of error, and associated functional problems.[2–6] Patient education about the appropriate use of the correction is especially important for persons with hyperopia. The correction often does not change visual acuity but reduces symptoms if used properly.

Hyperopia is defined as the condition in which parallel rays of light enter the eye and focus behind the retina when accommodation is relaxed.[7] Hyperopia can be corrected by a plus lens or by the patient's accommodation. Visual acuity is unaffected in hyperopia if the amount of hyperopia is low or if the patient's amplitude of accommodation is enough to neutralize the error. The effort of accommodation, however, may cause the patient to experience discomfort, particularly when performing near work, so that even low amounts of hyperopia may need to be corrected. High amounts of hyperopia decrease visual acuity, the decrease in acuity always being larger at near than it is at distance. High hyperopia that is not corrected at a young age can lead to unilateral or bilateral refractive amblyopia. Hyperopia is often associated with esophoria, esotropia, or strabismic amblyopia. These secondary binocular problems can be minimized or eliminated with correction of the refractive error.

Hyperopia changes little throughout life and is not associated with the kinds of pathologic changes that are seen with myopia. Typically,

most all children have hyperopia at 5 years of age, and their hyperopia decreases somewhat during childhood. The increases seen in
adolescents and adults with hyperopia are not really increases in hyperopia, but are increases in the amount of hyperopia manifested at
refraction as the amplitude of accommodation diminishes with age.[3,6,8]

Prescription Considerations and Guidelines

Adult Hyperopia

The most common type of hyperopic patient encountered by the optometrist is an adult with a low amount of facultative hyperopia. *Facultative hyperopia* is that which can be neutralized by the patient's
accommodation. Distance visual acuity is unaffected, and there are
usually no symptoms until the person reaches young adulthood, when
the person first experiences discomfort with near vision. The distance
refraction or some modification of it is then prescribed for use at near.
Patients can often see clearly with the prescription at distance but because they experience symptoms only with close work, they are advised to use the lenses for near vision only. As the patient ages, more
hyperopia becomes manifest on refraction, and the near prescription
is increased. At some point, patients notice that they can see clearly
with the prescription for distance as well as for near and eventually
start to wear the lenses full time.

For most adults between the ages of 20 and 40 years with low to
moderate hyperopia who have not worn glasses before, a prescription
is indicated if the patient has asthenopic symptoms. Visual acuity is
rarely affected at distance unless there is also uncorrected astigmatism. If patients do have any loss of acuity, it is only at near or the loss
is greater at near than at distance. The loss of acuity occurs when the
patient's amplitude of accommodation is not sufficient to neutralize
the hyperopic error. The prescription given to the patient is for use at
near and can be the amount of plus found on a routine noncycloplegic distance refraction. The patient is advised to wear the lenses for
near vision.

When a patient is given the distance refractive correction for use at
near, the demand on accommodation for near work becomes the
same as it is with emmetropia. Without correction, the patient would
have to accommodate for the working distance and for the amount of
hyperopia. With correction, the patient needs to accommodate only
for the distance of the object and not for hyperopia. There is little
need for cycloplegic refraction in patients 20 to 40 years of age who
have near symptoms, unless the prescription based on the noncycloplegic refraction does not alleviate the symptoms.

Some persons with hyperopia need no correction or need only a
partial correction. If visual acuity is adequate for their needs at both

distance and near, if they have no asthenopic symptoms, and if they do not show functional problems when they accommodate to neutralize their hyperopia, patients do not need a prescription.[4,9,10] The amount of hyperopia does not determine the decision to prescribe or not to prescribe; the patient's symptoms should be used as the optometrist's guide to prescription.

Partial hyperopic prescriptions should be given to adult patients with clinically significant amounts of latent hyperopia. Latent hyperopia is suspected when patients have an amplitude of accommodation less than expected for their age, when patients are esophoric at distance through the manifest plus refraction, when the results of the binocular balance show considerably more plus than the monocular subjective refraction, when static retinoscopy shows considerably more plus than the subjective refraction, or when the patient's plus prescription does not reduce the patient's near symptoms.

Cycloplegic refractions should be performed whenever latent hyperopia is suspected.[2,11,12] Prescription of the full cycloplegic refraction for distance is not recommended for adult patients, because it is likely to blur the patient's distance vision. Augsberger[2] recommends prescription of the full cycloplegic refraction and use of a cycloplegic agent such as cyclopentolate four times per day to help the patient overcome the accommodative spasm and adapt to the lenses. The results of the cycloplegic refraction can sometimes be prescribed for use at near, or the manifest refraction can be prescribed for distance with plus add that will decrease the patient's near symptoms.

Prescription of as much plus as possible without blurring the patient's distance vision and giving additional plus for near in the form of a bifocal if the patient's symptoms so warrant is recommended. Patients who are given a partial prescription should be seen for follow-up examinations about 6 weeks after they begin wearing their partial prescription and every 3 months after that until their refractive findings are stable and their symptoms have been alleviated. As they begin to relax their accommodation, patients manifest more plus on noncycloplegic refraction, and the prescription can be changed accordingly. It is essential to teach the patient about the need for wearing the lenses full time to reduce accommodation and ultimately to reduce the symptoms. These patients with latent hyperopia are often reluctant to wear glasses because their vision is as good without correction as it is with correction. They often express a fear that they will become dependent on their glasses if they start to wear them. The optometrist needs to anticipate these fears and remind the patient that glasses can be prescribed for comfort as well as for improvement in vision.

Accommodation and Vergence

The discomfort experienced by persons with uncorrected hyperopia is most often caused by the accommodative effort needed to neutralize the hyperopic error. It also can be caused by the effort to maintain binocularity. Many persons with uncorrected hyperopia have esophoria at both distance and at near and must use their supply of negative fusional vergence to maintain single binocular vision. Correction of the hyperopia decreases the esophoria, decreases the demand on negative fusional vergence, and often relieves the patient's symptoms.

Patients with a high accommodative convergence/accommodation (AC/A) ratio have a larger amount of near esophoria (or perhaps near esotropia) than distance esophoria, which can be decreased with the prescription of additional plus at near. Careful measurement of the phoria is essential in the decision about how much plus to prescribe for near vision. Although plus is good, more plus is not necessarily better. Esotropia with uncorrected hyperopia can become exotropia with corrected hyperopia if too much plus is prescribed.[10,13,14] This situation can be avoided if the optometrist measures the phoria through different amounts of plus and prescribes the amount that brings the patient's eyes closest to orthophoria.

Persons with exophoria and hyperopia who need correction because their amplitude of accommodation is not sufficient to compensate for the hyperopia may need vision therapy to increase their positive fusional vergence before plus is prescribed. Phorias and vergence should be measured through the tentative prescription as well as the habitual prescription before the final prescription is determined.

Adults with anisometropic hyperopia and refractive or strabismic amblyopia often present for routine examinations with no symptoms or present for an eye examination when they start to experience symptoms of presbyopia. These patients often have a history of not wearing glasses that were prescribed for them as children, or they say they "cheated" to pass vision screening tests and have never undergone a complete eye examination. These patients are often very aware of the difference in acuity in their two eyes and of their lack of depth perception. They sometimes ask if their depth perception can be improved or if anything can be done to improve the visual acuity in the poorer eye. Some of these patients have vocational needs for good visual acuity or good stereopsis. These patients should be given protective eyewear (polycarbonate lenses in a safety frame) with the appropriate prescription for their "good" eye.

Severity of the Hyperopia

The amount of hyperopia found at manifest refraction or at cycloplegic refraction is only a starting point in the determination of a prescription for hyperopia. The Orinda Study[15] recommended complete eye examinations for children with 1.50 diopters of hyperopia found during a vision screening. This is often the minimum amount of plus that optometrists consider prescribing for both children and adults. Ciner recommended correction of hyperopia of 2.00 diopters or more in pediatric patients to prevent refractive amblyopia and binocular problems.[10] However, even lower amounts of hyperopia should be corrected if the patient has asthenopic symptoms, esophoria or esotropia, or accommodation-convergence anomalies.

First-Time and Habitual Lens Wear

A patient's previous prescription should not necessarily be a factor in prescription for hyperopia. Some persons with hyperopia who have been given a low plus prescription, stop wearing their glasses and find that they no longer experience symptoms. These patients can discontinue wearing their glasses and are relieved to hear that they will not damage their eyes by doing so. These patients should be told that there may come a time when they will again need to wear their glasses but that if they are comfortable without glasses they do not need to wear them.

For patients with presbyopia, the optometrist should always use caution in increasing plus prescriptions for distance. Despite an improvement in visual acuity on a Snellen chart, some patients with hyperopia and presbyopia report blurry vision at distance through a plus prescription. The proposed distance plus prescription should always be trial framed for these patients, and the patients should look out the window as well as at the Snellen chart to be sure they are comfortable with their vision. For patients who find the full prescription blurs their vision (despite reading 20/15 on the Snellen chart), the optometrist reduces the plus in 0.25 diopter steps until the patient says his or her vision is clear. Visual acuity should be 20/40 or better at distance for all patients who drive. Changes of not more than 1.00 diopter are generally more successful than larger changes. Milder and Rubin recommended that all increases in plus prescriptions routinely be 0.25 diopter less than the manifest refraction at 6 meters.[5]

Pediatric Hyperopia

Decisions about prescriptions for adults with hyperopia are largely based on the patient's symptoms. These same principles can be used in prescription for children, but prevention of amblyopia and strabismus must also be considered, particularly for children younger than 6 years. In addition, few children younger than 6 years are able to articulate their visual needs and describe their symptoms. Bilateral refractive amblyopia can occur in persons with hyperopia with an error as low as 2.50 diopters. Unilateral refractive amblyopia can develop in persons with anisometropic hyperopia with as little as 1.00 diopter difference between the eyes.[16]

Persons with hyperopia at risk for the development of refractive amblyopia should receive full correction at an early age. However, because refractive error is changeable in children younger than 3 years, the prescription should not be given to the patient until the optometrist has found the same results at several visits.[10] Once the prescription has been determined, parents must be educated about the child's need to wear the glasses full time to ensure proper development of the child's vision. The optometrist should see patients younger than 6 years for follow-up examinations every 3 months to monitor visual acuity and to check on the patient's compliance with wearing the glasses.

Cycloplegic refractions are useful in determining a prescription for a young patient. Children have a much larger amplitude of accommodation and more active accommodation than do adults.[12] It is often difficult for children to maintain distance fixation for the duration of static retinoscopy and subjective refraction. A cycloplegic refraction is indicated for children when latent hyperopia is suspected, when there is esophoria or esotropia, or when there is decreased visual acuity that is not corrected with refraction. Children younger than 6 years are susceptible to refractive amblyopia, esotropia, or strabismic amblyopia if they have a moderate or high amount of uncorrected hyperopia or if they have a high AC/A ratio and even a small amount of hyperopia. Generally 1% cyclopentolate is sufficient to produce cycloplegia in children, though some authors recommend the use of atropine, particularly for children with esotropia.[12,13] Full cycloplegic correction is recommended for children with hyperopia and refractive amblyopia followed by amblyopia therapy if vision has not improved with full-time use of glasses.[10,11,13]

With children older than 6 years, the visual needs must be considered in decisions about the appropriate prescription. Children usually will not wear a prescription that blurs their vision. Older children who are in school have more critical visual needs than young children and are not able to wear a plus prescription that blurs their distance vision. Children show remarkable logic about glasses: if the glasses improve things, they wear them; if not, they balk at wearing glasses. A post-cycloplegic refraction is as important in older children with critical visual needs as it is in adults. If the full cycloplegic prescription noticeably blurs the patient's distance vision, the full plus prescription found at noncycloplegic refraction is given with additional plus in the form of an add for near if there is clinically significant esophoria, esotropia, or latent hyperopia.

When determining a prescription without cycloplegia, the optometrist needs to find the maximum plus prescription. It is common to find more plus on binocular balance than on monocular subjective refraction in persons with hyperopia. Other noncycloplegic methods of refraction that manifest maximum plus include the fog technique, the Borish delayed subjective refraction, the subjective through base-in prism, and binocular refraction with the American Optical (Southbridge, Massachusetts) Vectograph slide. These techniques are described in other publications.[1]

Persons with accommodative esotropia need a plus prescription that decreases the esotropia as much as possible. They need addition plus at near if the cover test shows a larger esotropia at near than at distance. Caution must be used in determining the add, since too much plus can produce exotropia.[10,13,14] The prescription should be for full-time wear. Parents need to be told that the child's eyes will be straight only when the child is wearing the glasses and that they will see the eyes turn when the child removes the glasses.

Progressive addition lenses can be used by older children who have mastered the use of bifocal lenses. For younger children, an executive or flat-top bifocal set at mid pupil is recommended so that the child cannot avoid using the near segment.

Children with low amounts of hyperopia have good visual acuity without correction but need a prescription if they have asthenopic symptoms. The minimum amount of plus that optometrists consider prescribing for children is often 1.50 to 2.00 diopters.[10,15,16] However, children with low amounts of hyperopia may have asthenopic symptoms that warrant a prescription. Just as with adults with low amounts of hyperopia, the patient's symptoms are the most important factor in deciding on a prescription. Sometimes children need low plus lenses for a few years and then find that they are comfortable without glasses. Use of the glasses can be discontinued as long as the patient is comfortable and is not at risk for development of amblyopia.

Spectacle Lens and Frame Design

Prescriptions for low amounts of hyperopia can be made in just about any frame and of any ophthalmic material. Patients with higher prescriptions should be counseled to keep the eye size of the frame small and to use lightweight and high index lenses. When bifocals are needed, progressive addition lenses can be used by older children and adults. Young children should be given an executive or flat-top bifocal with the segment set at mid pupil.

Contact Lenses

Fewer persons with hyperopia wear contact lenses than do persons with myopia, because persons with hyperopia often wear their glasses only parttime. Most persons with hyperopia have a low to moderate error that does not affect distance visual acuity. Patients with high hyperopia should be counseled about the cosmetic benefits of contact lenses.[13] Ciner recommended contact lenses for persons with hyperopia greater than 5.00 diopters.[10] Press and Moore recommended contact lenses for patients with anisometropia of 3.00 diopters or more.[13] Patients who wear their plus prescription full time are more motivated to wear contact lenses than those who wear their prescription for near only or for part-time wear. Patients who engage in athletics also may want to consider contact lenses, even if they wear the lenses only part-time. The amount of plus given to a contact lens wearer with hyperopia is greater than the amount in spectacles because of lens effectivity.

Case Studies of Hyperopia

Patient C.P.

History: C.P., a 40-year-old firefighter, presented for a routine eye examination on the advice of his internist, who noticed that C.P. had never undergone an eye examination. The patient reported that his vision was good for both distance and near and denied any symptoms when reading. C.P.'s general health was good; he had no allergies and was taking no medications. The family history was unremarkable.

Clinical Findings		6 m	40 cm
Habitual VA:	OD	20/15	20/20
	OS	20/15	20/20
Cover Test:		ortho	4^ΔXP′
Stereo Acuity at 40 cm:	20 seconds (Randot)		
Retinoscopy:	OD	+0.50 DS	
	OS	+0.50 DS	
SRx:	OD	+0.75 DS (20/15)	
	OS	+0.75 DS (20/15)	

Phorometry (w/SRx):	6 m	40 cm
Phoria	1^ΔEP	2^ΔXP′
NRA/PRA		+1.75/–2.00

Trial Frame: The subjective finding was trial framed, and C.P. was asked to compare his near vision and comfort with and without the prescription. C.P. reported that things looked and felt the same both with and without the prescription.

Assessment
1. Facultative hyperopia OU
2. Normal binocular vision

Treatment Plan
1. Rx: None at this time
2. Patient education: C.P. was advised to return for a routine eye examination in 2 years or sooner if he experienced any asthenopic symptoms, particularly when performing near work.

Discussion
The discussion of this case study is included with that of the following case study.

Patient K.W.

History: K.W., a 39-year-old bus driver, presented for an eye examination with a chief complaint of discomfort when reading. She had experienced this discomfort for the past 6 months. She also reported that she was having difficulty seeing road signs when driving at night. K.W. could not remember when she had last undergone an eye examination, and she had never worn glasses. K.W.'s general health was good, she was taking no medications, and she had no allergies. Further personal and family history was unremarkable.

Clinical Findings		6 m	40 cm
Habitual VA:	OD	20/20	20/40
	OS	20/15	20/40
Cover Test:		ortho	4$^\Delta$EP′
Stereo Acuity at 40 cm:	20 seconds (Randot)		
Retinoscopy:	OD	+0.75 DS	
	OS	+0.75 DS	
SRx:	OD	+0.75 DS (20/15)	
	OS	+0.75 DS (20/15)	

Phorometry (w/SRx):	**6 m**	**40 cm**
Phoria	ortho	2$^\Delta$XP′
NRA/PRA		+1.75/−1.00

Trial Frame: The subjective finding was trial framed and the patient was asked to compare her near vision and comfort with and without the prescription. The patient reported that things looked clear with the prescription and felt more comfortable with glasses, particularly for reading. She also said that her vision was as clear at distance with the prescription as it was without the lenses.

Assessment
1. Facultative simple hyperopia OU
2. Normal binocular vision

Treatment Plan
1. Rx: OD +0.75 DS
   OS +0.75 DS
2. Lens Design: Single vision resin lenses
3. Patient Education: The glasses were to be worn for all near work and for distance vision as needed. K.W. was advised to return for a routine examination in 2 years.

Discussion
Although both C.P. and K.W. had the same refractive error and were the same age, one of them had symptoms and the other did not. K.W.

described discomfort at near, and she had decreased visual acuity at near. C.P. had no symptoms and no loss of visual acuity at distance or at near. The prescription was trial framed for C.P. to give him an opportunity to see how his eyes would feel with his refractive error corrected, but because the patient did not notice a difference with the lenses, a prescription was not written. It is not necessary to correct a refractive error in the absence of decreased visual acuity and in the absence of symptoms. K.W. showed a clear need for a prescription and responded positively to the trial framing. It is possible that K.W. had symptoms because she had more latent hyperopia than C.P. A cycloplegic refraction was not performed, however, because the manifest refraction seemed to alleviate K.W.'s symptoms. As each of these patients becomes older and the amplitude of accommodation diminishes, any latent hyperopia they have will become manifest.

Patient E.W.

History: E.W., a 38-year-old computer systems analyst, presented for a routine eye examination. He reported clear, comfortable vision but said that vision with his left eye had always been poorer than with his right eye. E.W. said that he wanted glasses if they would improve his depth perception for hockey and golf. Glasses had been prescribed for E.W. several times between the ages of 7 and 25 years. E.W. rarely wore the glasses because he felt nauseated when he wore them and because they did not improve his vision. E.W. reported that his general health was good; he was taking no medications and had no allergies. The family history was unremarkable.

Clinical Findings		**6 m**	**40 cm**
Habitual VA:	OD	20/20	20/20
	OS	20/300	20/800
	OS	20/300 (w/pinhole)	
Cover Test:		ortho	ortho'
Retinoscopy:	OD	+0.50 DS	
	OS	+6.25 −3.00 × 30	
SRx:	OD	+1.00 DS (20/20)	
	OS	+6.25 −3.00 × 30 (20/200, 20/200 w/PH)	

Assessment
1. Facultative hyperopia OD
2. Compound hyperopic astigmatism (with-the-rule) OS
3. Anisometropia (5.25 diopters at 30° and 2.25 diopters at 120°)
4. Refractive amblyopia OS

Treatment Plan

1. Rx: OD   +1.00 DS
         OS   +1.00 DS (balance lens)
2. Lens Design: Polycarbonate single vision lenses in a safety frame
3. Patient Education: E.W. was advised to wear the lenses full time to decrease the risk of injury to his better eye. A re-examination in 1 year was recommended.

Discussion

If E.W. had received an appropriate correction and been counseled about wearing his glasses as a child, the vision in his left eye would be considerably better than 20/200. At the age of 38 years, full correction of the amblyopic eye would not improve E.W.'s ability to function, because the vision in the left eye was best corrected to 20/200. In addition, E.W. had a history of difficulty adjusting to glasses. Because E.W. did not have a "spare eye" it was important to protect the good eye. Glasses with polycarbonate lenses in a safety frame were prescribed with the manifest refraction for the right eye, and a balance lens was prescribed for the left eye.

Patient W.W.

History: W.W., a 31-year-old computer programmer, presented for an eye examination with a chief complaint of distance blur through his habitual (current) glasses (HRx), which were first prescribed when he was 29 years of age. W.W. reported that he wore his glasses when working at the computer and for driving at the end of the day. His general health was good. He was taking no medications and had no allergies. His father had a history of high blood pressure. Further family history was unremarkable.

Clinical Findings		6 m	40 cm
Habitual VA:	OD	20/25	20/20 with −0.50 −1.00 × 80
	OS	20/25	20/20 with −0.75 −0.75 × 90
Cover Test (w/HRx):		ortho	ortho'
Stereo Acuity at 40 cm:	40 seconds (Randot)		
Retinoscopy:	OD	−0.75 −1.00 × 90	
	OS	−0.75 −0.75 × 90	
Monocular SRx:	OD	−0.50 −1.00 × 80 (20/20)	
	OS	−0.75 −0.75 × 90 (20/20)	
Binocular Balance:	OD	+2.00 −1.00 × 80 (20/20)	
	OS	+0.75 −0.75 × 90 (20/20)	

During the monocular subjective on the left eye, W.W. reported that he could read the letters but they were blurring in and out. Surprisingly, the binocular balance showed that W.W. did not have myopia at all but rather had moderate hyperopia. A cycloplegic refraction was performed 40 minutes after the instillation of two drops of 1% cyclopentolate in each eye, 5 minutes apart.

Cycloplegic Refraction:
OD +1.50 –1.00 × 80 (20/20)
OS +1.00 –0.75 × 90 (20/20)
Ocular Health, Tonometry and Visual Fields: Normal OU

W.W. was scheduled for a postcycloplegic examination 1 week later.

Postcycloplegic Refraction:
OD +1.75 –1.00 × 80 (20/20)
OS +1.00 –0.75 × 90 (20/20)
Trial Frame: Because this was a change of +2.25 D in the right eye and a change of +1.75 D in the left eye (relative to the patient's HRx) and because W.W. had reported distance blur, the response to trial framing was most important. The postcycloplegic prescription was trial framed, and W.W. walked around the office and looked out the window. He reported that things looked blurry. The sphere was reduced in 0.25 diopter steps in each eye until W.W. said his vision was clear. The prescription that W.W. reported as clear and comfortable was the following:
OD +1.25 –1.00 × 80
OS +0.50 –0.75 × 90

Assessment
1. Latent hyperopia OU (compound hyperopic astigmatism OD and mixed astigmatism OS)
2. Slightly reduced stereo acuity; otherwise normal binocular vision

Treatment Plan
1. Rx: OD +1.25 –1.00 × 80
   OS +0.50 –0.75 × 90
2. Lens Design: Single vision resin lenses
3. Patient Education: W.W. was instructed to wear the lenses full time and was advised to return for re-examination in 3 months.

Discussion
W.W. had an unusual case of adult hyperopia in which a cycloplegic refraction was clearly indicated after the manifest refraction showed an unexpected result when compared with the previous prescription. Although advised to return in 3 months, W.W. returned 6 months later. He reported that he was wearing his glasses only when his eyes were tired because he did not want to become dependent on the

glasses. W.W.'s distance visual acuity was 20/30 in each eye with the plus correction given to him at the previous visit. The binocular balance was similar to the refraction found at his previous visit. The refraction findings at re-examination were as follows:

OD   +2.00 –1.00 × 80 (20/20)
OS   +1.00 –0.75 × 90 (20/20)

W.W. was again instructed to wear his glasses full time rather than only when his eyes were tired. A considerable amount of time was spent on patient education with W.W. The optometrist explained that W.W. needed to wear his glasses to prevent his spasm of accommodation. W.W. was told that he would not become dependent on his glasses but would be more comfortable and would see better if he wore them consistently. W.W. was told to return for a re-examination in 1 year. Once W.W. had been wearing his glasses consistently and his accommodation stabilized, the prescription could be increased. Modification of the prescription power would become easier as W.W. aged and his amplitude of accommodation decreased.

Patient C.K.

History: C.K., a 6-year-old girl, presented for her first eye examination after failing a school screening. She said she had no vision complaints, and her parents had not noticed any vision problems. C.K.'s general health was good. She was taking no medications and had no known allergies. The family history was unremarkable.

Clinical Findings		6 m	40 cm
Habitual VA:	OD	20/40	20/40
	OS	20/50	20/40
Cover Test:		4^ΔEP	10^ΔEP'
Stereo Acuity at 40 cm:	100 seconds (Randot)		
Keratometry:	OD	43.37/41.75 at 90° (against-the-rule)	
	OS	43.87/42.25 at 90° (against-the-rule)	
Retinoscopy:	OD	+5.25 –1.00 × 90 (20/25)	
	OS	+4.75 –0.75 × 90 (20/25)	

Cycloplegic Refraction (40 minutes after the instillation of two drops of 1% cyclopentolate 5 minutes apart):

OD   +6.75 –1.00 × 90 (20/25)
OS   +6.25 –0.75 × 90 (20/25)

Postcycloplegic Refraction 1 Week Later:

OD   +5.25 –1.00 × 90 (20/25)
OS   +4.75 –0.75 × 90 (20/25)

Trial Frame: Both the cycloplegic and the postcycloplegic refraction findings were trial framed. C.K. reported that her vision was the same without correction as it was with the postcycloplegic finding and that her distance vision was blurred with the cycloplegic finding. C.K. further stated that she did not think she needed glasses at all.

Assessment
1. Compound hyperopic astigmatism (against-the-rule) OU
2. Slight refractive amblyopia OU

Treatment Plan
1. Rx: OD   +5.25 –1.00 × 90
        OS   +4.75 –0.75 × 90
2. Lens Design: Polycarbonate single vision lenses in a small frame
3. Patient Education: The importance of wearing the glasses full time was emphasized to C.K.'s mother. C.K. was instructed to return for a follow-up examination in 3 months. At her follow-up examination 3 months later, C.K. reported that she had been wearing her glasses full time and that she now felt that her vision was much better with the glasses than without them. C.K.'s mother reported that she had a hard time getting C.K. to remove her glasses.

Clinical Findings During Follow-up Examination
Habitual VA:

		6 m	40 cm
	OD	20/30	20/25 with +5.25 –1.00 × 90
	OS	20/25	20/20 with +4.75 –0.75 × 90

Cover Test (w/Rx): ortho   ortho′
Stereo Acuity at 40 cm: 70 seconds (Randot)
Retinoscopy: OD   +5.75 –1.25 × 90
                OS   +5.25 –1.25 × 90
SRx: OD   +5.75 –1.25 × 90 (20/25)
                OS   +5.25 –0.75 × 90 (20/25)

Discussion
Because C.K. showed more manifest hyperopia, the prescription was increased by 0.50 diopter in each eye. She was scheduled to be seen again in 6 months. A near add was not indicated for C.K. because her phoria was ortho at near through her distance prescription and she was comfortable with it. If C.K. continued to manifest more hyperopia in the future, her prescription would likely be increased. The cover test would also be carefully monitored, and an add would be prescribed if clinically significant esophoria were found. When C.K.'s vision and binocular findings were stabilized, the possibility of contact lenses would be discussed with her mother.

Patient A.C.

History: A.C., a 9-year-old girl in fourth grade, had been wearing single vision glasses for constant wear since the age of 6 years. She reported that her vision with her glasses was good at distance and near but that she was uncomfortable when reading for more than 20 minutes. A.C.'s general health was good. She was taking no medications and had no allergies. The family history was unremarkable.

Clinical Findings		6 m	40 cm
Habitual VA:	OD	20/20	20/20 with +5.00 DS
	OS	20/20	20/20 with +4.75 DS
Cover Test (w/Rx):		ortho	15ᐞAET'
Stereo Acuity at 40 cm (w/Rx): No response (Randot)			
Retinoscopy:	OD	+5.00 DS	
	OS	+5.00 DS	
SRx:	OD	+5.00 DS (20/20)	
	OS	+4.75 DS (20/20)	

Cover Test at 40 cm			
(w/SRx):		**w/+2.00 D add**	**w/+2.50 D add**
		ortho'	5ᐞAXT'

Assessment
1. Simple hyperopia OU
2. Accommodative alternating esotropia

Treatment Plan
1. Rx: OD   +5.00 DS +2.00 D add
   OS   +4.75 DS +2.00 D add
2. Lens Design: Polycarbonate executive bifocal lenses set with the segment height at mid pupil to ensure that the patient would use the add for all near work.
3. Patient Education: A.C. was instructed to wear the glasses full time and to use the bifocal segment for all near work. The purpose of the segment was explained to the patient and the parent. A follow-up examination in 3 months was recommended.

Discussion
A.C. had high hyperopia with accommodative esotropia but was wearing a correction only for the hyperopia. Accommodative esotropia can be corrected with additional plus at near. The first add to try is +2.50 D in an attempt to completely relax the accommodative response at a viewing distance of 40 centimeters. However, this proved to be too much plus and caused consecutive exotropia. The add was

reduced to +2.00 D, which gave A.C. a near phoria of ortho. Before the final prescription is written, the cover test should be repeated to ensure that in solving one problem, a new problem is not created, for example, opposing phoria.

Patient J.S.

History: J.S., a 12-year-old boy in seventh grade, presented for an eye examination with a chief complaint of blurred vision at near. He reported that he read several hours per day and especially enjoyed magazines and newspapers. J.S. reported that his symptoms are more acute when reading newspaper or magazine print than when reading school books. J.S.'s last eye examination had been at 6 years of age. The refraction at that time was +0.25 D OU. He had never worn glasses. J.S.'s general health was good. He was taking no medications and had no allergies. The family history was unremarkable.

Clinical Findings		6 m	40 cm
Habitual VA:	OD	20/20	20/20
	OS	20/20	20/20
Cover Test:		4$^\Delta$EP	6$^\Delta$EP′
Stereo Acuity at 40 cm:	20 seconds (Randot)		
Retinoscopy:	OD	+1.00 –0.75 × 90	
	OS	+0.75 DS	
Monocular SRx:	OD	+1.00 –0.75 × 90 (20/20)	
	OS	+0.50 DS (20/20)	
Binocular Balance:	OD	+1.50 –0.75 × 90 (20/20)	
	OS	+1.25 DS (20/20)	

Phorometry (w/SRx):	6 m	40 cm
Phoria	ortho	ortho′

Trial Frame: The binocular balance was trial framed, and J.S. reported that his eyes felt much more comfortable with the lenses than without, particularly when reading. He also said his vision was clear across the room through the glasses.

Assessment
1. Facultative hyperopia OU (compound hyperopic astigmatism OD and simple hyperopia OS)
2. Normal binocular vision

Treatment Plan
1. Rx: OD +1.50 –0.75 × 90
   OS +1.25 DS

2. Lens Design: Single vision polycarbonate lenses
3. Patient Education: J.S. was instructed to wear the glasses during school and to use them for reading and all other near work. A follow-up visit in 3 months was scheduled.

J.S. returned for the follow-up visit in 3 months. He reported that he was wearing his glasses all day in school and that his vision was clear and comfortable with the glasses. His visual acuity with correction was 20/20 in each eye at distance and at near, and his refraction was unchanged.

Discussion

J.S.'s uncorrected visual acuity was 20/20 at distance because he used his accommodation to neutralize his hyperopia. At 12 years of age, according to Donder's table,[1] J.S. should have an amplitude of accommodation of 12 to 13 diopters. This is certainly sufficient to neutralize a hyperopia of 1.25 diopters at distance and to accommodate 3.75 diopters for reading at 40 centimeters. J.S. most likely experienced symptoms caused by the esophoria present at distance and near when his vision was uncorrected. When the hyperopia was corrected, J.S. did not have to accommodate at distance and his esophoria decreased to ortho. With correction at near, the accommodative demand was reduced from 3.75 diopters to 2.50 diopters and again the phoria decreased to ortho. Although J.S. had a low amount of hyperopia, the correction was necessary to make him comfortable, and he adjusted well to wearing glasses. Because the near prescription was based on the distance refraction, J.S. was still able to see clearly at distance and did not need additional plus for near.

Summary

In adults with low hyperopia and asthenopic symptoms, one should prescribe the distance refraction for near. As their amplitude of accommodation decreases with age, patients begin to manifest more plus on refraction and the prescription can be increased. Gradually, the patient will need lenses full time and will need an add when presbyopia occurs.

Patients with large amounts of latent hyperopia and accommodative spasms need to wear their lenses on a consistent basis. They may need more plus at near than at distance and can be given bifocals or two pairs of glasses if the distance refraction for near use does not reduce the asthenopic symptoms.

Adults with low hyperopia that does not decrease visual acuity at distance or at near do not need a prescription of plus if they have no symptoms and no accommodative or convergence anomalies. The prescription should be demonstrated in a trial frame so these patients can decide whether or not they feel the prescription improves their comfort. Not every case of hyperopia necessitates correction. In low hyperopia, the patient's symptoms should dictate whether or not a prescription is needed.

Children younger than 6 years should undergo a full cycloplegic refraction when refractive amblyopia or esotropia is present. School-age children should be given maximum plus that does not blur distance vision. If esophoria or esotropia is present, the patient can be given a plus add for near. The add should be the amount of plus needed to maximize the alignment of the two eyes.

Children with a low amount of hyperopia and near symptoms can be given their distance refraction for use at near. This prescription can be increased as the patient's amplitude of accommodation decreases with age and as he or she begins to manifest more hyperopia on refraction.

Patients of any age are unlikely to wear lenses that blur their vision. If a patient needs more plus for near than that found at distance refraction, the correction should be provided in the form of a bifocal lens. Patient who have worn bifocals for a long period of time often manifest more hyperopia for distance; the distance prescription can then be increased and the bifocal eliminated.

Trial framing of proposed prescriptions, modification of the prescription on the basis of the patient's response to the trial, and appropriate patient education should lead to success in prescription of lenses for persons with hyperopia.

References

1. Carlson NB, Kurtz D, Heath DA, Hines C. *Clinical Procedures for Ocular Examination.* Norwalk, Conn: Appleton & Lange, 1990:12,94–103.

2. Augsburger A. Hyperopia. In: Amos JF, ed. *Diagnosis and Management in Vision Care.* Boston: Butterworth-Heinemann, 1987:101–119.

3. Borish I. *Clinical Refraction.* 3rd ed. Chicago: Professional Press, 1970:115–122.

4. Michaels DD. *Visual Optics and Refraction.* St. Louis: Mosby, 1985:471–472.

5. Milder B, Rubin ML. *The Fine Art of Prescribing Glasses Without Making a Spectacle of Yourself.* Gainesville, Fla: Triad Scientific, 1991:17–30.

6. Grosvenor T. *Primary Care Optometry.* New York: Professional Press, 1989:332.

7. Schapero M, Cline D, Hofstetter HW. *Dictionary of Visual Science.* Philadelphia: Chilton, 1968:335–336.

8. Grosvenor T, Flom MC. *Refractive Anomalies Research and Clinical Applications*. Boston: Butterworth-Heinemann, 1991:121–127,131–144.

9. Sloane AE. *Manual of Refraction* 2nd ed. Boston: Little, Brown, 1970:39–40.

10. Ciner EB. Management of refractive error in infants, toddlers, and preschool children, In: Scheiman MM, ed., *Problems in Optometry: Pediatric Optometry.* 1990;2:394–419.

11. Scheiman M, Wick B. *Clinical Management of Binocular Vision.* Philadelphia: Lippincott, 1994:85,490–508.

12. Rosner J, Rosner J. *Pediatric Optometry.* 2nd ed. Boston: Butterworth-Heinemann, 1990:147–149.

13. Press LJ, Moore BD, *Clinical Pediatric Optometry.* Boston: Butterworth-Heinemann, 1993:242–251,253–263.

14. Beneish R, Williams F, Polomeno RC, Little JM. Consecutive exotropia after correction of hyperopia. *Can J Ophthalmol* 1981;16:16–18.

15. Blum HL, Peters HB, Bettman JW. *Vision Screening for Elementary Schools, the Orinda Study.* Berkeley & Los Angeles: University of California Press, 1968:21–35.

16. Ingram RM. Refraction as a basis for screening children for squint and amblyopia. *Br J Ophthalmol* 1977;61:8–15.

Case Study Exercises

For each case study, determine the diagnosis and develop a treatment plan. The clinical questions provided for each case may assist you by highlighting important aspects of the case.

Patient R.B.

History: R.B., a 36-year-old nursing student, presents with a chief complaint of tired eyes after 20 minutes of near work. He has never worn glasses and underwent his last eye examination 10 years ago because he had a piece of metal in his right eye. R.B.'s general health is good. He is taking no medications and has no known allergies. R.B.'s maternal grandmother had cataracts. Further history was unremarkable.

Clinical Findings		**6 m**	**40 cm**
Habitual VA:	OD	20/20	20/20
	OS	20/20	20/20
Cover Test:		ortho	6$^\Delta$EP′
Stereo Acuity at 40 cm:	20 seconds (Randot)		
Keratometry:	OD	42.00/42.50 at 90°	
	OS	42.75/43.00 at 90°	
Retinoscopy:	OD	plano sphere	
	OS	plano sphere	
Monocular SRx (SRx 1):			
	OD	+0.75 DS (20/20)	
	OS	+0.50 DS (20/20)	
Binocular Balance (SRx 2):			
	OD	+1.00 DS (20/15)	
	OS	+1.00 DS (20/15)	

Phorometry (w/SRx 2):	**6 m**	**40 cm**
Phoria	ortho	3$^\Delta$XP′
NRA/PRA		+2.25/–2.50

Clinical Questions
1. Given the patient's symptoms, what type of refractive error do you expect to find?
2. Given the patient's uncorrected visual acuity, what type of refractive error do you expect to find?
3. How much total refractive astigmatism do you expect based on the keratometry readings?

4. Why is there a difference between the near phoria measured with the cover test and the near phoria measured by phorometry?
5. Does this patient need a prescription? Why or why not?

Patient T.C.

History: T.C., a 7-year-old boy, is undergoing his first eye examination after failing a vision screening at his pediatrician's office. T.C. reports no problems with his eyes and is doing well in school. His parents have not noticed any eye problems. T.C.'s general health is good. He is taking no medications and has no known allergies. The family history is unremarkable.

Clinical Findings		6 m	40 cm
Habitual VA:	OD	20/30	20/40
	OS	20/30	20/40
Cover Test:		4$^\Delta$EP	8$^\Delta$EP'
Stereo Acuity at 40 cm:	100 seconds (Randot)		
Keratometry:	OD	44.50/45.00 at 90°	
	OS	45.00/45.50 at 90°	
Retinoscopy:	OD	+7.00 DS (20/40)	
	OS	+7.00 DS (20/40)	
SRx:	OD	+6.50 DS (20/30, same with pinhole)	
	OS	+6.50 DS (20/30, same with pinhole)	

Because the visual acuity is not correctable to 20/20 with the subjective refraction, a cycloplegic refraction is performed 40 minutes after the instillation of two drops of 1% cyclopentolate in each eye, 5 minutes apart.

Cycloplegic Refraction:
        OD   +6.50 DS (20/30)
        OS   +6.50 DS (20/30)
Ocular Health, Tonometry and Visual Fields: Normal OU

T.C. is scheduled for a postcycloplegic refraction in 1 week. The postcycloplegic refraction yields no change from the previous cycloplegic refraction with the same 20/30 best corrected acuities.

Clinical Questions
1. What type of refractive error do you predict for this patient on the basis of the uncorrected visual acuity?
2. Why is the patient's visual acuity still reduced with the correction?
3. What would you prescribe for this patient? Should he wear the lenses for near only or full time? Why or why not?
4. How soon should this patient undergo a follow-up examination?
5. What is the prognosis for this patient?

Patient A.L.

History: A.L., an 8-year-old girl in second grade, is seen for a routine examination. She reports no problems and is progressing well in school. Her parents have not noticed any vision problems. A.L.'s general health is good, she is taking no medications, and she has no known allergies. The family history is unremarkable.

Clinical Findings		6 m	40 cm
Habitual VA:	OD	20/15	20/20
	OS	20/15	20/20
Cover Test:		ortho	2ᐃXP'
Stereo Acuity at 40 cm:	20 seconds (Randot)		
Keratometry:	OD	43.00/43.50 at 90°	
	OS	42.87/43.37 at 90°	
Retinoscopy:	OD	+1.25 DS	
	OS	+1.25 DS	
Monocular SRx (SRx 1):			
	OD	+0.75 DS (20/15)	
	OD	+0.50 DS (20/15)	
Binocular Balance (SRx 2):			
	OD	+1.00 DS (20/15)	
	OS	+1.00 DS (20/15)	

Phorometry (w/SRx 2):	6 m	40 cm
Phoria	ortho	6ᐃXP'

Clinical Questions

1. Given the patient's uncorrected visual acuity, what type of refractive error do you expect to find?
2. Does this patient need a prescription? Why or why not?
3. What would be an appropriate treatment plan for this patient?

Patient R.G.

History: R.G., a 59-year-old truck driver, is seen for a routine examination because his wife thinks he needs one. He has been wearing glasses for reading only since the age of 42, and reports no vision problems. R.G. has been taking hydrochlorothiazide for high blood pressure for 6 years. He last saw his internist 1 month before his eye examination and reports that his blood pressure is under good control with medication. R.G. has no known allergies. Further personal and family history is unremarkable.

Clinical Findings

		6 m (w/o Rx)	40 cm (w/Rx)
Habitual VA:	OD	20/100 (20/25 w/PH)	20/40 with +3.00 DS
	OS	20/50 (20/20 w/PH)	20/25 with +2.50 DS
Cover Test (w/HRx):		ortho	8ΔXP′
Keratometry:	OD	45.00/45.50 at 90°	
	OS	44.75/45.25 at 90°	
Retinoscopy:	OD	+1.50 DS	
	OS	+1.00 DS	
SRx:	OD	+1.75 –0.25 × 90 (20/15)	
	OS	+1.00 –0.25 × 90 (20/15)	

Tentative Add at 40 cm: +2.25 D (20/20)

NRA/PRA with a +2.25 D Add: +0.75/–0.75

Range of Clear Vision (w/+2.25 D add): 25 to 50 cm

Ocular Health, Tonometry and Visual Fields: Normal OU

Clinical Questions
1. Given the patient's history and uncorrected visual acuity, what type of refractive error do you expect to find? Can you predict the amount of refractive error from the uncorrected acuity?
2. Does this patient need a distance prescription? Why or why not?
3. What form of spectacle lenses would you recommend for this patient?

4   Astigmatism

Robert C. Capone

A Case Study of Astigmatism

History: K.H., a 36-year-old electronics technician presented for an eye examination stating that he "needed glasses" because his had been lost. K.H. reported headaches, eyestrain, and sensitivity to light. He stated that he had to squint to see things more clearly but that doing so gave him a headache. K.H.'s last examination had been 2 years before the current visit, and he had been wearing glasses off and on since he was 7 years of age.

K.H. reported that at 7 years of age his very first pair of glasses "drove him crazy" and that he refused to wear them. With that correction, K.H. reported that he saw telephone poles tilted instead of straight, that the floor seemed warped, that he felt nauseated, and that all these symptoms were aggravated when he was moving. K.H. also reported that his current prescription gave him the same feelings and was the reason he wore the glasses only occasionally. The patient and family ocular and medical histories were unremarkable. The patient took no medications and had no known allergies.

Clinical Findings		6 m	40 cm
Habitual Visual			
Acuity (VA):	OD	20/50 (20/20 w/pinhole)	20/50
	OS	20/50 (20/20 w/pinhole)	20/50
Cover Test (w/o Rx):		ortho	ortho'

Amplitude of Accommodation (w/o Rx): OD 4.00 diopters, OS 4.00 diopters, OU 5.00 diopters
Near Point of Convergence (NPC): 12.5 cm
Stereo Acuity (w/o Rx): 50 seconds (Randot)

Keratometry:	OD	45.00/43.00 at 90° (against-the-rule)
	OS	45.00/43.50 at 90° (against-the-rule)
Retinoscopy:	OD	+0.25 –3.00 × 90
	OS	plano –2.75 × 90
Subjective Refrac-tion (SRx):	OD	+0.50 –3.00 × 90 (20/20)
	OS	–0.25 –2.75 × 90 (20/20)

Phorometry (w/SRx):	**6 m**	**40 cm**
Phoria	ortho	4^{Δ}XP′
Base-in (BI) vergence	X/8/5	12/22/12
Base-out (BO) vergence	10/19/11	14/20/10

Ocular Health, Tonometry and Visual Fields: Normal OU
Trial Frame: The subjective refraction data were trial framed. K.H. reported that although objects appeared clear, the walls and floor seemed tilted. The tilting appeared to worsen when K.H. walked around. A second trial framing with the following prescription was performed:

$$+0.25 –2.50 × 90 \text{ OD}$$
$$–0.50 –2.00 × 90 \text{ OS}$$

This prescription was more comfortable for K.H. and provided 20/20 acuity OU without the symptoms of spatial distortion.

Assessment
1. Mixed astigmatism (against-the-rule) OD and compound myopic astigmatism (against-the-rule) OS
2. Slightly reduced stereo acuity due to reduced uncorrected visual acuity; otherwise, binocular vision normal

Treatment Plan
1. Rx: OD +0.25 –2.50 × 90
   OS –0.50 –2.00 × 90
2. Lens Design: Single vision resin lenses (CR-39) were fabricated in a small eye size with a close vertex distance.
3. Patient Education: The patient was instructed to wear the glasses full time and return in 3 months for a follow-up visit consisting of a visual acuity measurement and an assessment of his symptoms. The prognosis for this patient was good.

Symptoms and Signs of Astigmatism

K.H.'s case illustrates many of the common signs and symptoms associated with a moderate to high amount of astigmatism, such as headaches, eyestrain, squinting, and problems adapting to a spectacle prescription.

Although astigmatism greater than 2 diopters accounts for a small percentage (2% to 6%) of all cases of astigmatism, these cases are encountered by all practitioners, and many can be quite challenging to manage.[1] The typical patient reports blurry vision at distance and near as well as asthenopic symptoms such as headaches, eyestrain, browache, and burning and irritated eyes.[2-6] Much of the asthenopia is caused by prolonged squinting, which leads to muscle fatigue.

Patients who have had a previous prescription are likely to report that it took them a long time to get used to their glasses. This is because of the spatial distortion these patients experience. Symptoms such as seeing flat surfaces (for example, walls and floors) as warped and vertical lines (for example, telephone poles and stop signs) as tilted are commonly associated with an initial spectacle correction for astigmatism.[2-7] Most patients adapt to these distortions in a matter of days to weeks. However, some patients have great difficulty adapting and continue visiting their optometrists. Many of these unhappy patients arrive with a shopping bag full of glasses that have failed to give them clear, comfortable vision. If one takes a logical approach to each patient and listens carefully, many cases of astigmatism can be managed quite easily.

Prescription Considerations and Guidelines

Age of the Patient

Many important issues to consider are specific to age. For young children, the consensus of practitioners has been to administer the full correction.[8,9] The question remains, however, at what age to write a prescription for a given patient. Should one prescribe glasses if large amounts of astigmatism are detected at 1 or 2 years of age? The answer is no. Astigmatism changes during the early years of life and probably reaches adult levels by 3 to 5 years of age.[10,11] Because the early years are critical in visual development, high degrees of astigmatism should be fully corrected to allow for normal visual development and the prevention of meridional amblyopia, a form of refractive amblyopia.[12]

A good general rule for patients older than 2 years, as outlined by Ciner,[13] is to examine the patient every 3 months for three visits. If the amount of astigmatism has remained stable, it is time to prescribe glasses for full-time wear. The visual cortex has great plasticity during the early years, and providing the sharpest retinal image possible (with the full prescription) will prevent the development of amblyopia. Young children do exceptionally well with the full prescription (determined by cycloplegic refraction) and adapt quite easily.[14,15]

If the patient is an older child (age 10 through the teens) whose vision has not been corrected, the full prescription still should be given. However, because of reduced plasticity and increased visual demands, the patient may experience more symptoms due to spatial distortion when first wearing the new glasses. Therefore, it is imperative to provide careful patient and parent education about the importance of wearing the glasses full time to facilitate adaptation.

The issues with adult patients are quite different. The options are a full prescription versus a partial prescription. Many authors and practitioners subscribe to the philosophy of giving the full prescription as a first option.[3-5] Practitioners who do administer a full prescription to an adult must be careful to teach the patient about the spatial distortions that may be perceived when the patient first wears the glasses. The patient should be told that the adaptation period may last a few days to weeks.

A conservative approach with many adult patients is to administer a full prescription to patients who have symptoms with their old glasses and seem open to a change in prescription. This is especially true if the patient notices improvement in visual acuity with modified cylinder power or axis. In addition, a patient who has a relaxed, "laid back" personality might also be open to change and may adapt easily to a new prescription.

A partial prescription for patients who are anxious, highly sensitive, critical, or meticulous is often a better option than to prescribe the full cylinder prescription determined during the refraction. These patients are notorious for having unsuccessful results with a full prescription because they are "driven crazy" by the spatial distortions. Patients who have a history of frequent changes of prescription or have large amounts of astigmatism at oblique axes (which cause the maximum amount of spatial distortion) respond better to a partial than to a full prescription.

As adults age, they experience symptoms of a reduced amplitude of accommodation, that is, presbyopia. By the time presbyopia is manifested, most patients have already adapted to some form of distance prescription and have successfully dealt with many of the issues related to a spectacle correction. To minimize the risk of failure, many factors must be taken into consideration before one administers a new prescription to patients with emerging presbyopia.

One such factor is the nearpoint cylinder axis, which is often different from that found at distance in patients with moderate to high astigmatism. Failure to take the difference in cylinder axis between distance and near viewing into consideration will likely result in an unsuccessful reading prescription. The base curve of a spectacle lens is a second factor to consider in contemplating bifocal lenses for a patient with presbyopia. The bifocal lens will likely have a base curve different from that of the patient's habitual single vision lens. Failure to consider the difference in base curve can lead to failure due to changes in spatial distortion. Third, for patients who require an anisometropic prescription, consideration must be given to the possible vertical imbalance at near point with bifocal lenses. One must also remember that older adults are prone to degenerative and systemic disease. Many have undergone ocular surgeries, and their vision must be stabilized before a permanent prescription is administered.[16,17]

Severity of Astigmatism

The higher the degree of astigmatism, the greater is the difficulty the patient will have accepting a correction. Higher amounts of astigmatism are usually associated with higher amounts of spherical component ametropia (that is, hyperopia and myopia). The astigmatism in many of these cases is congenital; however, some may be associated with abnormalities of the cornea, such as keratoconus or pterygia, which may cause severe distortion of the cornea with resultant irregular astigmatism.[2,3,17]

Among children who have a large hyperopic as well as an astigmatic component, the incidence of amblyopia depends on the patient's age when the first prescription was administered. This is true because at no place in object space is a patient with uncorrected vision able to see clearly. If there is a large myopic and astigmatic component, the eye has a far point in real space, although it may be close to the patient's face, where the object is almost clear. Therefore, in myopic astigmatism there is a risk of amblyopia, though the risk is smaller than if the patient has compound hyperopic or mixed astigmatism.

The type of astigmatism (that is, with-the-rule, against-the-rule, or oblique) is as important a consideration in the prescription of lenses as is the amount of astigmatism. Patients who have with-the-rule or against-the-rule astigmatism have the advantage of being able to squint to try to improve their vision. Through the combined effect of lid pressure and the pinhole effect, the visual acuity of a squinting patient will improve a small amount. However, a patient with oblique astigmatism is at a disadvantage, because squinting has minimal effect and because correction at an oblique axis will produce maximal spatial distortion.[18–20]

For patients with high degrees of irregular astigmatism, regardless of the cause, spectacle correction is only a compromise. Better results may be obtained with rigid contact lenses or refractive surgical procedures.

First-Time and Habitual Lens Wear

If a patient is happy with a habitual prescription and has acceptable visual acuity with it, the optometrist should not change the prescription. Optometrists who do change a prescription in such circumstances may regret doing so. However, if visual acuity, stereopsis, or comfort decreases with the habitual prescription and the practitioner can demonstrate to him- or herself and to the patient that these factors improve with the new cylinder power or axis, a change should be considered.

For adults wearing glasses for the first time, trial framing the proposed prescription to see how sensitive the patient is to spatial distortion is desirable. The decision to reduce the prescription to facilitate adaptation can then be made. The question is then, "How do you know how much to cut or modify the prescription?" This question can be answered by use of any of the following options.

1. *Reduce cylinder power and maintain spherical equivalent.* This option places the "circle of least confusion" of the remaining astigmatic interval on the retina, allowing for the clearest vision possible. For every 0.50 diopter decrease of minus cylinder, the sphere must be increased –0.25 D. This modification provides relatively clear vision and decreases the spatial distortion associated with the meridional magnification that occurs with high cylindrical prescriptions.

2. *Underprescribe the cylinder initially and then increase cylinder power over time.* This option is best tried in a trial frame with the sphere lens from the refraction in place and the axis of the cylinder set to that required. Cylinder power is added 0.25 diopter at a time until acceptable vision is obtained without the symptoms of spatial distortion.[21] This technique may be more successful than the spherical equivalent when one deals with corrections of large amounts of anisometropia.

3. *Use the old cylinder axis and modify the cylinder power.* For a patient who has had problems adapting to changes in cylinder axis, this is a very good option. Using the old cylinder axis, one performs a Jackson crossed-cylinder (JCC) power refinement and then adjusts the spherical component until the patient achieves best visual acuity.

4. *Move the axis toward 90° or 180°.* This technique is based on the fact that adaptation occurs more rapidly for cylinders that are close to axis 90° or 180°. In fact, the earlier literature mentions this option frequently. Because this technique creates residual astigmatism due to obliquely crossed cylinders, it is not recommended.

Accommodation and Vergence

In cases of bilateral astigmatism, optical correction can enhance fusional vergence to overcome small amounts of fusional anomaly at distance. With correction, the sharpened retinal image also facilitates the accuracy of accommodation for near objects with resultant changes in accommodative vergence.[22] The effects of image sharpness, improved accuracy of accommodation, and fusional vergence justify consideration of a prescription for astigmatism in the initial management of binocular anomalies. Caution must be used, however, to make sure an analysis of binocularity is performed with the new prescription. If binocularity is not analyzed, a patient with a previously asymptomatic, uncorrected vision problem who suppressed the use of an eye, may experience diplopia or strabismus.[22,23]

The optometrist must take special care when prescribing cylinder for a patient who has high astigmatism in one eye and has a spherical refractive error in the other eye. Patients with this type of correction might experience symptomatic anisophoria when they look away from the optical centers of the lenses. In this situation, a partial prescription may be more appropriate, but only if the patient is not a child and amblyopia is not a factor.

When the cylinder power is high, it is wise to measure the axis and power of the cylinder for near as well as for distance vision. Failure to adjust the axis for near may cause decreased near acuity due to the excyclotorsion that occurs when the eyes converge to view a nearpoint object. When the eyes experience excyclotorsion for near vision, the cylinder axes become misaligned with the principal meridians of the eye and the patient reports blurred vision at near.

To measure the change in cylinder axis and power at nearpoint, the optometrist performs a binocular refraction with the patient fusing on nearpoint text.[4,24,25] The left eye can be fogged with a retinoscopy lens and the right eye subjected to refraction with a JCC axis and power refinement. The procedure is repeated with the right eye fogged and the JCC axis and power refinement performed on the left eye. A distance-to-near difference in cylinder axis of greater than 5° or cylinder power greater than 0.75 diopter may produce problems if not corrected. The most effective solution is to prescribe a separate pair of reading glasses with the appropriate nearpoint sphere, cylinder axis, and power.

Meridional Aniseikonia

Because cylindrical lenses have a different power in each meridian, the magnification (or minification) of objects varies in each meridian. Although a patient with astigmatism in one eye will only rarely find the induced distortion disturbing, a patient with astigmatism in both eyes is likely to be deeply troubled by the problems of stereoscopic distortion that occur because of meridional aniseikonia.[26,27] This is especially true if the two lenses differ in their power by 1.00 diopter cylinder or more in corresponding meridians. Fortunately, many of these disturbing effects are minimized with adaptation and the use of appropriate spectacle lens designs.

Spectacle Design

One can specify a number of spectacle design features when ordering a prescription. The appropriate spectacle design will minimize the spatial distortion experienced by patients with moderate to high astigmatism. Features such as vertex distance, lens thickness, and base curves are successful because of their effects on the total magnification of the lens. Some features should be modified initially, and some are special features that may be varied if initial attempts at correction, as described next, are unsuccessful.

1. *Frame size.* The frame size should be as small as possible. The smaller the lens diameter, the less is the peripheral distortion that will be perceptible to the patient. As the eye rotates away from the optical centers, more induced prism is encountered. Greater distortion is often associated with larger eye sizes.

2. *Vertex distance.* Choose a frame that will keep the distance between the ocular surface of the spectacle lens and the cornea (vertex distance) to a minimum. The closer a lens is to the entrance pupil of the eye, the less is the spatial distortion experienced by the patient. This is one of the reasons contact lenses work so well for many patients for whom use of spectacles has not worked.

Another way to alter vertex distance is to specify a one-third to two-thirds bevel design. This type of design places the lens bevel closer to the front surface of the lens and shortens the vertex distance. This works particularly well with high minus prescriptions.[28] Decreasing the vertex distance in a positive lens leads to a decreased power magnification. Conversely, decreasing the vertex distance in a minus lens leads to an increased power magnification.

3. *Use of minus cylinder lenses.* The use of minus cylinders in spectacle prescriptions is common because their effect on shape magnification minimizes distortion. When the front surface of a spectacle lens is spherical, the magnification associated with the base curve and center thickness will be the same in all meridians, producing a change in retinal image size that is uniform throughout the image. The converse is true of a plus cylinder lens that has a toric front lens surface.

4. *Placement of the optical centers.* Accurate placement of the optical centers is extremely important, since it is only as the eyes rotate away from the optical centers that problems arise. This is especially important for patients who are given a prescription for a separate pair of reading glasses. Consideration should be given to dropping the optical centers 2 to 3 mm below the frame center to simulate the reading posture. Some patients drop their head when they read; for them, only an accurate near pupillary distance is warranted.

5. *Index of refraction of the lens material.* When ordering a spectacle prescription, one should consider the material used. This is especially true if the specifications of the existing prescription are duplicated. As many practitioners are aware, changing to a higher index material allows use of thinner lenses with decreased center thickness. At the same time, a higher index lens has a flatter base curve. These two factors, that is, flatter base curves and decreased center thickness, affect the shape magnification and ultimately total magnification. Practitioners should choose lens materials carefully.

Special Lens Design Considerations

If a patient is properly educated about spatial distortion and the practitioner has carefully followed the recommendations for lens design, most patients will adapt to their prescriptions in a few days to 2 weeks. However, if the patient continues to have problems, the practitioner may have to consider a change in base curve or center thickness or consider an iseikonic lens design.

Changes in base curve and center thickness alter spatial distortion by changing shape magnification and ultimately the total magnification of the lens. An increase in base curve results in an increase in the shape magnification of a lens. However, for prescriptions greater that –2.50 D, an increased base curve results in a decreased overall magnification, because an increased front curvature translates into an increased vertex distance. As center thickness increases, the magnification increases. Changes in the base curve and center thickness should not be made arbitrarily. Other texts and optical surfacing charts should be consulted to change these parameters to produce the desired magnification adjustments.

Use of iseikonic lens designs can be attempted, but such lenses are rarely used in general practice because of a lack of practitioner experience in designing them. These lenses often provide poor cosmesis and they are expensive. It also is difficult to find a laboratory capable of manufacturing these lenses. Therefore, before considering iseikonic lens designs, the practitioner should consider prescribing contact lenses. Contact lenses often eliminate the problems of meridional aniseikonia and provide comfortable binocular vision. For further information on designing iseikonic lenses, consult other sources dealing with the treatment of aniseikonia and bitoric spectacle lens design.[28–32]

Vocational and Avocational Considerations

When providing a prescription, it is important to consider the patient's occupational and vocational visual needs. Of course these will vary with all age groups and occupations. However, certain situations should be considered. A child wearing a prescription full time needs to have a sturdy frame and preferably polycarbonate lenses for eye protection. This is especially important for children involved in sports.

Teenagers and adults involved in sports often benefit a great deal from contact lenses. Contact lenses provide the ultimate benefit of a large peripheral field of view without distortion, allow clear vision, and present minimal magnification problems. Contact lenses may be of the spherical or toric design, depending on the amount of corneal toricity. If contact lenses are chosen, suitable safety eyewear also should be used.

Contact lenses are not an option for patients who work in a setting where they may be exposed to volatile fumes. This is because the fumes may become bound to the contact lens material, prolonging contact between the fumes and the eyes, which may result in corneal compromise.

Patients with presbyopia present an interesting challenge. For these patients with high astigmatism (for example, greater than 4 diopters), progressive addition lenses (PALs) are probably not a good option, because the inherent peripheral distortion in PALs combines with the distortion produced by the cylinder in the lenses.

Case Studies of Astigmatism

Patient C.D.

History: C.D., a 29-year-old college student, had difficulty with a new pair of "high index glasses" she received from her family eye doctor 1 month prior. She stated that when she wore the glasses everything seemed slanted and she felt "cross-eyed." She had tried to get used to the glasses for 1 month but had no luck and as a result got into an argument with her doctor. C.D. continued to wear her old glasses, which were scratched but did not make her "feel sick." C.D. stated that she had been wearing glasses since the age of 6 years and had no eye injuries or infections. The patient's ocular and medical history were remarkable for environmental allergies for which she took antihistamines as needed.

Current Habitual
Rx (HRx 1):   OD   −5.00 −3.50 × 160
                   OS   −5.00 −4.25 × 40

The lenses were made of 1.6 high index resin with an interpupillary distance (IPD) of 60 mm, a base curve of +2.50 D, and a center thickness of 1.5 mm.

Previous Habitual
Rx (HRx 2):   OD   −4.75 −3.00 × 160
                   OS   −5.00 −4.00 × 40

These lenses were scratched and made of hard resin (CR-39) with an IPD of 60 mm, a base curve of +4.50 D, and a center thickness of 2.2 mm.

Clinical Findings		**6 m**	**40 cm**
Habitual VA (w/HRx 1):	OD	20/20	20/20
	OS	20/20	20/20
Habitual VA (w/HRx 2):	OD	20/30^{+2}	20/25
	OS	20/25	20/25
Cover Test (w/HRx 2):		ortho	4$^\Delta$XP′

Amplitude of Accommodation (w/HRx's): 8.00 D OD, OS, OU
Stereo Acuity at 40 cm (w/HRx's): 25 seconds (Randot)

Keratometry:	OD	45.00/48.00 at 70° (with-the-rule)
	OS	45.00/49.00 at 130° (oblique)
Retinoscopy:	OD	−4.75 −3.25 × 160
	OS	−5.00 −4.50 × 40
SRx:	OD	−5.00 −3.50 ×160 (20/20)
	OS	−5.00 −4.25 × 40 (20/20)

Phorometry (w/SRx):	**6 m**	**40 cm**
Phoria	ortho	6$^\Delta$XP′
BI vergence	X/8/5	14/22/15
BO vergence	10/20/12	15/20/10
Negative Relative Accom-		
modation (NRA)/Positive		
Relative Accommodation (PRA):	+2.50/−2.00	

SRx at 40 cm:	OD	−5.00 −3.25 × 162
	OS	−5.00 −4.00 × 38

Trial Frame: The patient reported clear and comfortable vision with the subjective refraction data.

Assessment
1. Compound myopic astigmatism OU (with-the-rule OD and oblique OS)
2. Symptoms from the most current prescription (HRx 1) that were absent with the previous prescription (HRx 2) were most likely caused by a combination of the changes of base curve, center thickness, and lens material in the former from those of the latter.

Treatment Plan
1. Rx: OD −5.00 −3.50 × 160
      OS −5.00 −4.25 × 40
2. Lens Design: single vision resin lenses (CR-39) with a base curve of +4.50 D and center thickness of 2.2 mm

3. Patient Education: C.D. was informed of the reason for her symptoms with the newer prescription and that the changes of certain lens parameters to those of her previous prescription would likely eliminate those symptoms.

Discussion

This case demonstrates the powerful effect of changes in lens parameters in some patients. A change to a higher index material necessitates a flatter base curve and decreased center thickness. These two factors ultimately translate into changes in shape magnification and therefore can result in problems with adaptation. With high prescriptions in particular, it is usually advisable to maintain the habitual lens parameters if possible, especially if the patient has no symptoms. In this case, using hard resin lenses with a duplicate base curve and center thickness eliminated the patient's symptoms of perception of slanting of the environment and "crossed-eyes."

Patient F.R.

History: F.R., a 5-year-old boy, presented for an eye examination after failing a school screening. F.R.'s mother stated that she had noticed her son squinting to see the television and that when she read him stories at night, he placed his face very close to the book. F.R.'s medical and ocular history and that of his family were unremarkable. F.R. took no medications and had no known allergies.

Clinical Findings		6 m	40 cm	
Habitual VA:	OD	20/60 (20/30 w/PH)	20/100	
	OS	20/60 (20/30 w/PH)	20/100	
Cover Test:		4$^\Delta$EP	10$^\Delta$EP'	
Stereo Acuity at 40 cm:	100 seconds (Randot)			
Keratometry:	OD	44.00/47.00 at 90° (with-the-rule)		
	OS	44.25/47.25 at 90° (with-the-rule)		
Retinoscopy:	OD	+1.50 −2.50 × 180		
	OS	+1.50 −2.75 × 180		
SRx:	OD	+1.50 −2.50 × 180 (20/30, 20/30 w/PH)		
	OS	+1.50 −2.75 × 180 (20/30, 20/30 w/PH)		

Phorometry (w/SRx):	6 m	40 cm
Phoria	2$^\Delta$EP	4$^\Delta$EP'
BI vergence	Not performed because of patient's inability to cooperate	
BO vergence	Not performed because of patient's inability to cooperate	

Because he was physically fatigued, F.R. was asked to return on another day for a cycloplegic refraction. The results were as follows:

SRx (w/
  cycloplegia):   OD   +3.00 −3.50 × 180 (20/30)
                 OS   +3.00 −3.75 × 180 (20/30)

Assessment

1. Mixed astigmatism (with-the-rule) OU
2. Decreased visual acuity OU secondary to refractive amblyopia

Treatment Plan

1. Rx: OD   +3.00 −3.50 × 180
         OS   +3.00 −3.75 × 180
2. Lens Design: A sturdy plastic frame with polycarbonate lenses
3. Patient Education: F.R. was instructed to wear the glasses full time and return in 3 months for a visual acuity recheck.

Discussion

This case is fairly typical of children who usually present as a result of failing a school screening or because a parent has noticed something peculiar about his or her child's visual behavior. As indicated earlier, squinting allows for improved clarity of vision because of the pinhole effect and changes in corneal curvature with lid pressure. In the case of this child, holding reading material closer allowed a larger image size to fall on the retina and allowed visual targets to be more easily differentiated.

F.R.'s visual acuities show that acuity in both eyes was decreased at near more than at distance, leading one to believe that there is a hyperopic component to his refractive error. Since pinhole acuities show improvement to 20/30, it is likely that refraction will yield only this acuity. At this point two possibilities could exist for the decreased vision: amblyopia or a pathologic condition.

An esophoric posture greater at near than at distance provides clues to the hyperopic component of the refractive error. Here the accommodative system tries to compensate for some of the uncorrected hyperopia and move the "circle of least confusion" closer to the retina; in the process, however, it drives the eyes into an esophoric posture.

The presence of an esophoria greater at near than that at distance should indicate the need for a cycloplegic refraction. During the cycloplegic refraction, more hyperopia was uncovered but there also was an unmasking of more astigmatism than was detected with the noncycloplegic refraction. In the presence of good ocular health, the patient's decreased acuity was attributed to refractive amblyopia.

At the follow-up visit, F.R.'s mother reported that her son no longer sat "on top of things" and had adjusted well to his glasses. In fact, he was so excited about wearing his glasses that he did not want to take them off at bedtime. Visual acuity with correction revealed 20/25^{+2} OD and OS and stereopsis of 30 seconds. The patient was being examined routinely and was 6 years of age at the follow-up visit. Visual acuity with glasses was 20/20 OD and OS one year after the initial evaluation, and F.R. was doing well in school.

Patient C.S.

History: C.S., a 35-year-old real estate broker, presented for examination stating that she had been having a great deal of difficulty with her reading vision after receiving a new prescription from another practitioner. She had continued to go back to the practitioner to complain, but he stated that C.S. "had to get used to them." One month later, C.S. continued to have problems. She stated that her new prescription worked well for driving but she read better with her old prescription.

Current Rx (HRx 1):	OD	−6.50 −4.00 × 180
	OS	−4.00 −3.75 × 30
Previous Rx (HRx 2):	OD	−6.00 −3.75 × 15
	OS	−4.25 −3.25 × 20

C.S. had worn glasses since age 6. Her medical history was unremarkable. Family history was remarkable for hypertension and thyroid dysfunction. C.S. took no medications and was allergic to codeine and substances containing ephedrine.

Clinical Findings		6 m	40 cm
Habitual VA (w/HRx 1):	OD	20/20	20/30^{-2}
	OS	20/20	20/30^{-2}
Habitual VA (w/HRx 2):	OD	20/30^{+2}	20/25^{-1}
	OS	20/25	20/25^{-1}
Cover Test (w/HRx's):		ortho	3$^{\Delta}$XP′

Amplitude of Accommodation (w/HRx's): OD 5.00 diopters, OS 5.00 diopters, OU 6.00 diopters
NPC: 7.5 cm
Stereo Acuity at 40 cm (w/HRx's): 25 seconds (Randot)

Keratometry:	OD	44.25/48.00 at 90° (with-the-rule)
	OS	44.00/47.25 at 120° (with-the-rule)
Retinoscopy:	OD	−6.25 −4.00 × 180
	OS	−4.25 −3.50 × 030
SRx1 (6 m):	OD	−6.50 −4.00 × 180 (20/20)
	OS	−4.00 −3.75 × 030 (20/20)
SRx2 (40 cm):	OD	−6.00 −4.75 × 015 (20/20)
	OS	−3.75 −4.00 × 020 (20/20)

Phorometry:	6 m (w/SRx1)	40 cm (w/SRx2)
Phoria	ortho	4$^\Delta$XP'
Gradient phoria (+)		8$^\Delta$XP'
BI vergence	X/7/3	12/20/11
BO vergence	9/17/9	16/20/12

Assessment

1. Compound myopic astigmatism OU (with-the-rule)
2. Anisometropia (2.50 diopters)
3. Shift in axis of correcting cylinder at near point secondary to excyclotorsion OU

Treatment Plan

1. Distance Rx: OD −6.50 −4.00 × 180
                 OS −4.00 −3.75 × 30
2. Near Rx: OD −6.00 −4.75 × 15
                OS −3.75 −4.00 × 20
3. Lens Design: Small diameter hard resin (CR-39)single vision lenses with one-third to two-thirds bevel for the near prescription.
4. Patient Education: The need for two separate prescriptions resulting from the cylinder axis shift from distance to near was explained to C.S. She understood the reason for her decreased acuity at near with the distance prescription.

Discussion

Solving a case like this is a great accomplishment. The history discloses findings related to new glasses and problems at near point. The effects of excyclotorsion at near are magnified in a patient with high astigmatism secondary to the narrow tolerance for a shift in axis. There can be not only a shift in axis but also, as was illustrated, a change in sphere and cylinder power. This case also demonstrates the fact that the previous practitioner failed to recognize that he created a problem at near point when he prescribed the new prescription.

Patient R.U.

History: R.U., a 14-year-old high school student, presented with decreased vision in her right eye at distance and near and good vision in her left eye. She stated that she had a pair of glasses that was prescribed 2 years ago but did not like to use them because they made her "sick." She reported that when she wore the glasses objects seemed slanted and she felt as if she were falling. R.U.'s medical and ocular history and that of her family were unremarkable. R.U. took no medications and had no known allergies.

Clinical Findings		6 m	40 cm
Uncorrected VA:	OD	20/80	20/80
	OS	20/20	20/20
Habitual VA:	OD	20/30^{+2}	20/30 with +1.00 −3.50 × 070
	OS	20/20	20/20 with +0.50 DS
Cover Test (w/HRx):		ortho	6$^{\Delta}$XP′

Amplitude of Accommodation (w/HRx): OD 9.00 diopters, OS 11.00 diopters, and OU 11.00 diopters

Stereo Acuity at 40 cm(w/HRx): 40 seconds (Randot)

Keratometry:	OD	46.50/43.00 at 70° (against-the-rule)
	OS	43.00/43.50 at 90° (with-the-rule)
Retinoscopy:	OD	+1.50 −3.75 × 070
	OS	+0.75 DS
SRx:	OD	+1.00 −3.50 × 070 (20/30^{+2})
	OS	+0.50 DS (20/20)

Phorometry (w/SRx):	6 m	40 cm
Phoria	ortho	6$^{\Delta}$XP′
BI vergence	X/7/3	12/21/12
BO vergence	9/18/10	16/20/10
NRA/PRA		+2.50/−2.25

Trial Frame: The following prescription with the correcting cylinder in the right eye reduced by 1.50 diopters from the subjective data with the spherical equivalent maintained was provided in a trial frame.

OD +0.25 −2.00 × 70 (20/40^{+2})
OS +0.50 DS (20/20)

Although this prescription produced less slanting of objects, the patient was still bothered by the blurred vision in her right eye.

Assessment
1. Mixed astigmatism (against-the-rule) OD and simple hyperopia OS
2. Meridional aniseikonia
3. Decreased visual acuity OD secondary to meridional amblyopia

Treatment Plan
1. No change of the spectacle prescription at present
2. Patient Education: The diagnoses and symptoms were explained to R.U and her parents. R.U. was instructed to return for a contact lens evaluation and fitting. The visual acuity of the right eye would be monitored after the contact lens fitting.

Discussion
This case demonstrates the extreme difficulty patients encounter when trying to adapt to a prescription that contains a large cylindrical cor-

rection in one eye and a spherical correction in the other eye. Because the patient had normal binocular vision, stereoscopic distortion was manifested from the meridional aniseikonia of her spectacles. Reducing the cylindrical correction in the right eye while maintaining the spherical equivalent reduced the perception that objects slanted. However, the prescription also led to a decrease in acuity that was perceptible to the patient.

Because the patient had no contraindications to contact lens wear, a soft toric lens was fitted, which gave her 20/25 acuity (with difficulty) in her right eye. The left eye was left without correction. This patient was very happy not only with improved acuity and no distortion but also with good cosmesis.

Patient R.C.

History: R.C., a 28-year-old server in a restaurant, presented for an examination stating that she had been having difficulty seeing road signs, especially at night. She had not seen flashing lights or floating objects or experienced diplopia. Her hobbies included dancing and aerobics. R.C.'s ocular history was unremarkable except that this was her first eye examination. Her medical history was unremarkable. R.C.'s family medical history was remarkable for diabetes, hypertension, and heart disease (mother). The patient took no medications and had no known allergies.

Clinical Findings		6 m	40 cm
Habitual VA:	OD	20/25 (w/difficulty)	20/25 (w/difficulty)
	OS	20/200 (20/30 w/PH)	20/200
Cover Test (w/o Rx):		4$^\Delta$XP	8$^\Delta$XP'

Amplitude of Accommodation (w/o Rx): OD 8.00 diopters, OS 5.00 diopters, OU 8.00 diopters

Stereo Acuity at 40 cm (w/o Rx): 200 seconds (Randot)

Keratometry:	OD	44.00/45.00 at 90° (with-the-rule)
	OS	44.00/47.75 at 135° (oblique)
Retinoscopy:	OD	plano −1.25 × 180
	OS	+1.25 −4.25 × 45
SRx:	OD	−0.25 −1.00 × 180 (20/20^{+2})
	OS	+1.00 −4.00 × 45 (20/25 with difficulty)

Phorometry (w/SRx):	6 m	40 cm
Phoria	ortho	4$^\Delta$XP'
BI vergence	X/8/5	9/18/10
BO vergence	10/20/11	10/16/10
NRA/PRA		+2.25/−2.00

Trial Frame: Trial framing of the subjective refraction data for 15 minutes produced clear vision. However, the patient was extremely sensitive to the spatial distortion. The correcting cylinder power was reduced (maintaining the spherical equivalent) until the patient was not sensitive to the distortion. This occurred with the following prescription:

OD $-0.25 -1.00 \times 180$ ($20/20^{+2}$, 20/20 at 40 cm)
OS $+0.25 -2.50 \times 45$ ($20/30^{-2}$, 20/30 at 40 cm)

A repeated stereo acuity measurement at 40 cm with this prescription was 40 seconds.

Assessment

1. Compound myopic astigmatism (with-the-rule) OD and mixed astigmatism (oblique) OS
2. Slight decrease in visual acuity OS secondary to meridional amblyopia

Treatment Plan

1. Rx: OD $-0.25 -1.00 \times 180$
          OS $+0.25 -2.50 \times 45$
2. Lens Design: Small diameter frame with short vertex distance and hard resin (CR-39) single vision lenses
3. Patient Education: Amblyopia and the need for a full-time prescription was explained to R.C. She was instructed to return 1 to 2 months after the prescription was dispensed for a follow-up visit to remeasure visual acuity.

Discussion

It is interesting how some patients have never noticed their loss of visual acuity when they cover an eye. In fact, R.C. was asked if she ever noticed that the vision in her right eye was better than that in her left eye, to which she replied no. She then was asked to alternately occlude each eye while looking at the acuity chart. She was amazed at the difference in her vision.

There are a few important points to emphasize in this case. First, the visual acuity in the left eye improved with a pinhole to 20/30. Therefore, the subjective refraction should result in that level of acuity or perhaps a small amount better. Second, without correction the patient has not only reduced stereo acuity (because of blur) but also an exophoria at distance and near. One should note that with best correction, not only the phoria decreases but also stereo acuity improves. These changes can be attributed to the improved visual acuity, which resulted in greater facility of the fusional vergence system.

Although this patient did not tolerate the spatial distortion of the full prescription, a partial prescription provided improved acuity, im-

TABLE 4.1 Patient Selection Guidelines for Prescription of Full or Partial Correction of Astigmatism

Age Group	Full Prescription	Partial Prescription
Children	• Young children who have large amounts of stable astigmatism • Children who demonstrate refractive amblyopia	• Not recommended
Adults	• Patients who have problems with their habitual prescription and seem open to a prescription change and have noticed an improvement with the new cylinder axis or power • Patients with a "laid back" personality	• Patients who are anxious, highly sensitive, critical, or meticulous • Patients who have a history of frequent change because of poor adaptation to distortion • Patients with large amounts of astigmatism at oblique axes

proved stereopsis, and comfortable vision. Because the patient did not have extensive visual demands and did not have severe symptoms, the prescription could have been given on an as-needed basis. However, the patient will likely adapt to future changes in cylinder power by wearing her glasses full time. She will also have a better appreciation of what she has been "missing" (that is, clear vision) if she wears her glasses full time.

Summary

The management of moderate to high astigmatism can be challenging because one must consider many factors before prescribing lenses for a patient. Factors such as the patient's age, severity of the effects of the refractive error on the functional system, and spectacle design are but a few of the important areas. Important clinical problems to consider include amblyopia, anisometropia, and meridional aniseikonia.

Because a great deal of a patient's difficulty occurs as a result of the spatial distortion produced by corrective lenses, care must be given to the consideration of a full as opposed to a partial prescription (Table 4.1). Judicious application of these guidelines should assist the clinician in making difficult management decisions.

References

1. Borish IM. *Clinical Refraction.* 3rd ed. Chicago: Professional Press, 1970:123–148.

2. Bartlett JD. Anisometropia and aniseikonia. In: Amos JF, ed. *Diagnosis and Management in Vision Care.* Boston: Butterworth-Heinemann, 1987:173–202.

3. Michaels DD. *Visual Optics and Refraction: A Clinical Approach.* 3rd ed. St. Louis: Mosby, 1985:457–483.

4. Milder B, Rubin ML. *The Fine Art of Prescribing Glasses Without Making a Spectacle of Yourself.* 2nd ed. Gainesville, Fla: Triad, 1991:93–118.

5. Ostfeld H. General considerations in prescribing. In: Edwards K, Llewellyn R, eds. *Optometry.* Boston: Butterworth-Heinemann, 1988:465–474.

6. Coffeen P, Guyton DL. Monocular diplopia accompanying ordinary refractive errors. *Am J Ophthalmol* 1988;105:451–459.

7. Guyton DL. Prescribing cylinders: the problem of distortion. *Surv Ophthalmol* 1977;22:177–188.

8. Press LJ. Prescribing and fitting children's eyewear. In: Press LJ, Moore BD, eds. *Clinical Pediatric Optometry.* Boston: Butterworth-Heinemann, 1993:253–263.

9. Baldwin WR. Refractive status of infants and children. In: Rosenbloom AA, Morgan MW, eds. *Principles and Practice of Pediatric Optometry.* 2nd ed. Boston: Butterworth-Heinemann, 1993:104–153.

10. Atkinson J, Braddick O, French J. Infant astigmatism: its disappearance with age. *Vision Res* 1980;20:891–893.

11. Mohindra I. Early treatment of anisometropic astigmatism. *Am J Optom Physiol Opt* 1977;55:479–484.

12. Tanlamai T, Goss DA. Prevalence of monocular amblyopia among anisometropes. *Am J Optom Physiol Opt* 1979;56:704–715.

13. Ciner EB. Management of refractive errors in infants, toddlers, and preschool children. *Probl Optom* 1990;2:394–419.

14. Mitchell DE, Freeman RD, Millodot M, Haegerstrom G. Meridional amblyopia: evidence for modification of the human visual system by early visual experience. *Vision Res* 1973;13:535–558.

15. Dobson V, Fulton A, Lawson-Sebris S. Cycloplegic refractions of infants and young children: the axis of astigmatism. *Invest Ophthalmol Vision Sci* 1984;25:83–87.

16. Bogan S, Simon JW, Krohel GB, Nelson LB. Astigmatism associated with adnexal masses in infancy. *Arch Ophthalmol* 1987;105:1368–1370.

17. Roy FH. *Ocular Differential Diagnosis.* 5th ed. Philadelphia: Lea & Febiger, 1993:734–735.

18. Burian HM, Ogle KM. Meridional aniseikonia at oblique axes. *Arch Ophthalmol* 1945;33:293–309.

19. Ogle KN, Madigan LF. Astigmatism at oblique axes and binocular stereoscopic spatial localization. *Arch Ophthalmol* 1945;33:116–127.

20. Everson RW. Perceptual distortion with oblique cylindrical magnification. *Optom Weekly* 1973:5:457–458.

21. Carlson NB. Case report: a large change in cylindrical correction in an adult patient. *N Engl J Optom* 1985;27:19–21.

22. Flom MC, Wick B. A model for treating binocular anomalies. In: Rosenbloom AA, Morgan MW, eds. *Principles and Practice of Pediatric Optometry.* 2nd ed. Boston: Butterworth-Heinemann, 1993:245–273.

23. Scheiman M, Wick B. *Clinical Management of Binocular Vision.* Philadelphia: Lippincott, 1994:82–103.

24. Milder B. Lady luck. *Surv Ophthalmol* 1976;20:347–349.

25. Rutstein RP, Eskridge JB. Effect of cyclodeviations on the axis of astigmatism (for patients with superior oblique paresis). *Optom Vision Sci* 1990;67:80–83.

26. Sorsby A, Leary GA, Richards MJ. The optical components in anisometropia. *Vision Res* 1962;2:43–51.

27. Berens C, Bannon RE. Aniseikonia: a present appraisal and some practical considerations. *Arch Ophthalmol* 1963;70:93–100.

28. Scheiman M, Wick B. *Clinical Management of Binocular Vision.* Philadelphia: Lippincott, 1994:543–577.

29. Linksz A, Bannon RE. Aniseikonia and refractive problems. *Int Ophthalmol Clin* 1965;5:515–534.

30. Rayner AW. Aniseikonia and magnification in ophthalmic lenses: problems and solutions. *Am J Optom Arch Am Acad Optom* 1966;43:617–632.

31. Brown RM, Enoch JM. Combined rules of thumb in aniseikonic prescriptions. *Am J Ophthalmol* 1970;69:118–126.

32. Good GW, Polasky M. Eikonic lens design for minus prescriptions. *Am J Optom Physiol Opt* 1979;56:345–349.

Case Study Exercises

For each case study, determine the diagnosis and develop a treatment plan. The clinical questions provided with each case may assist you by highlighting important aspects of the case.

Patient J.C.

History: J.C., a 5-year-old boy, presents for his first examination. His mother states that she had noticed that her son held things very close to see them and that occasionally it appeared that J.C.'s right eye turned toward his nose. The patient's ocular and medical history are unremarkable. The family history is remarkable for glasses (father at age 7) and hypertension (maternal grandmother). The patient takes no medications and has no known allergies.

Clinical Findings		6 m	25 cm
Habitual VA:	OD	20/400 (20/50 w/PH)	20/400
	OS	20/400 (20/50 w/PH)	20/400
Cover Test (w/o Rx):		8$^\Delta$EP	14$^\Delta$EP′
Stereo Acuity at 40 cm (w/o Rx): <500 seconds (Randot)			
Keratometry:	OD	37.00/41.00 at 40°	
	OS	37.25/42.25 at 135°	
Retinoscopy:	OD	+7.00 −4.00 × 130	
	OS	+8.25 −5.00 × 45	
SRx:	OD	+6.50 −4.00 × 130	
		(20/40, same with pinhole)	
	OS	+7.50 −5.00 × 45	
		(20/40, same with pinhole)	
Cover Test (w/SRx): 2$^\Delta$EP at 6 m and 6$^\Delta$EP′ at 40 cm			

Phorometry:	6 m	40 cm
BI vergence	Not performed because of patient's inability to cooperate	
BO vergence	Not performed because of patient's inability to cooperate	

Refraction (w/cycloplegia):

OD	+9.00 −4.50 × 130 (20/40)	
OS	+10.50 −5.50 × 45 (20/40)	

Cover Test (w/ cycloplegic Rx):	6 m	40 cm
	ortho	2$^\Delta$XP′

Clinical Questions

1. Why does this patient hold material close, as indicated in the history?
2. On the basis of the entering visual acuities alone what ametropia would be expected?
3. What type of ametropia would cause the patient's eyes to assume an esophoric posture?
4. Does the amount of astigmatism found with subjective refraction correlate with that found with keratometry and retinoscopy?
5. Why is the acuity still reduced with best correction from cycloplegia?
6. What is an appropriate treatment plan for this patient?

Patient D.A.

History: D.A., a 32-year-old electrical engineer presents for a routine eye examination. He reports no problems with his current prescription for distance and near. D.A.'s last eye examination was 3 years ago. The patient's ocular history is positive for glasses at the age of 5. Both his mother and father wear glasses, as do his siblings. The patient and family medical history is unremarkable. The patient takes no medications and has no known allergies.

Clinical Findings		6 m	40 cm
Habitual VA			
(w/HRx):	OD	20/20^{-2}	20/20 with −2.00 −4.00 × 130
	OS	20/20	20/20 with −1.00 DS
Cover Test (w/HRx):		ortho	8$^{\Delta}$XP′
Amplitude of Accommodation: 8.00 diopters OD, OS, OU			
Stereo Acuity at 40 cm (w/HRx): 25 seconds (Randot)			
Keratometry:	OD	43.25/47.25 at 40°	
	OS	42.00/42.50 at 90°	
Retinoscopy:	OD	−1.75 −4.50 × 130	
	OS	−1.75 DS	
SRx:	OD	−2.25 −4.50 × 130 (20/20^{+1})	
	OS	−1.25 DS (20/20^{+2})	

Phorometry (w/SRx):	6 m	40 cm
Phoria	ortho	8$^{\Delta}$XP′
BI vergence	X/8/5	14/22/12
BO vergence	10/20/12	18/20/17
Gradient phoria (+)		11 XP′

Clinical Questions

1. Considering the amount of astigmatism in the patient's prescription, how can one account for such good acuity in the right eye?
2. Why does this patient not experience spatial distortion?
3. Is the 8^Δ exophoria at near a concern?
4. What is an appropriate treatment plan for this patient?

Patient R.N.

History: R.N., a 36-year-old teacher, presents for examination with symptoms of a slight decrease in vision at distance and near over the last few months. The last eye examination was 5 years ago. The patient wears glasses full time and has worn glasses since the age of 7 years. He says that he "hated" his glasses when he was young because they made things "look weird." The patient and family ocular history is unremarkable. The patient and family medical history is unremarkable. The patient takes no medications and has no known allergies. His hobbies included fishing and working on cars.

Clinical Findings		6 m	40 cm
Habitual VA			
(w/HRx):	OD	20/30⁺²	20/30 with $+1.00 -3.50 \times 70$
	OS	20/30⁺²	20/30 with $+2.00 -5.00 \times 110$
Cover Test (w/HRx):		2^ΔEP	4^ΔEP'

Amplitude of Accommodation: 5.00 diopters OD, 5.00 diopters OS, 6.00 diopters OU

Stereo Acuity at 40 cm: 40 seconds (Randot)

Keratometry:	OD	41.00/38.50 at 70°
	OS	42.25/37.25 at 110°
Retinoscopy:	OD	$+1.75 -4.25 \times 70$
	OS	$+3.00 -6.00 \times 110$
SRx at 6 m:	OD	$+1.75 -4.00 \times 70$ (20/20)
	OS	$+3.00 -6.00 \times 110$ (20/20)

Phorometry (w/SRx):	6 m	40 cm
Phoria	ortho	ortho'
BI vergence	X/10/6	13/21/13
BO vergence	10/21/12	15/18/11
NRA/PRA		+2.50/−2.25

Trial Frame: Some spatial distortion noted with the subjective refraction data

SRx at 40 cm:	OD	$+1.75 -4.50 \times 69$
	OS	$+2.75 -5.75 \times 112$
Trial Frame Rx:	OD	$+1.50 -3.50 \times 70$ (20/20)
	OS	$+2.50 -5.00 \times 110$ (20/20)

Clinical Questions
1. Are the patient's symptoms suggestive of a change in prescription?
2. Does the esophoria on the cover test provide a clue to expected findings in the refraction?
3. Should the full prescription be given even if the patient has symptoms with use of a trial frame?
4. What is an appropriate treatment plan for this patient?

Patient E.P.

History: E.P., a 52-year-old cab driver, presents for an eye examination because his "glasses were all scratched." He also notices that his reading vision is not as good as it used to be and that his eyes tire easily after reading. E.P.'s hobbies included golf and reading novels. He reports that his last eye examination was 2 years ago and that his ocular history is positive for wearing glasses since the age of 7 years. E.P. reports that he never liked to wear his glasses as a child because they made everything look distorted to him, but he says that he was "blind" without the glasses. E.P. has no known medical problems. The family history is positive for hypertension and cancer. The patient takes no medications and has no known allergies.

Clinical Findings		**6 m**	**40 cm**
Habitual VA:	OD	20/30	20/30 with +4.25 −6.50 × 03
	OS	20/30^{-3}	20/30^{-2} with +5.25 −8.00 × 175
			+2.25 D add OU
Cover Test (w/HRx):		ortho	6$^{\Delta}$XP′

Amplitude of Accommodation: 3.00 diopters OD, OS, OU
Stereo Acuity at 40 cm (w/HRx): 70 seconds (Randot)

Keratometry:	OD	39.75/46.25 at 93°
	OS	39.50/47.25 at 87°
Retinoscopy:	OD	+4.50 −6.50 × 03
	OS	+5.50 −8.00 × 175
SRx:	OD	+4.75 −6.50 × 03 (20/20)
	OS	+5.75 −8.00 × 177 (20/20)

Tentative Add at 40 cm: +2.25 D (20/20)

Phorometry (w/SRx):	**6 m**	**40 cm (w/+2.25 D add)**
Phoria	ortho	6$^{\Delta}$XP′
BI vergence	X/6/3	14/22/14
BO vergence	8/16/8	16/20/10
NRA/PRA		+0.75/−0.50

Range of Clear Vision (w/+2.25 D add): 20 to 45 cm

SRx at 40 cm: The cylinder axes changed to 5° OD and 175° OS. The cylinder power did not change.

Ocular Health, Tonometry and Visual Fields: Normal OU

Clinical Questions

1. Is the patient's chief complaint consistent with the habitual visual acuities at distance and near?
2. Why does the patient have no symptoms with regard to spatial distortion considering the high cylinder correction?
3. Why is there a slight change of the axis when the subjective refraction is performed at 40 centimeters?
4. Would a 2° change of the axis for the left eye cause distortion?
5. What is an appropriate treatment plan for this patient?

5 Anisometropia

Douglas K. Penisten

A Case Study of Anisometropia

History: D.P., a 6-year-old boy, presented for his first eye examination. He stated that "My eyes get tired when I'm reading." His mother reported she noticed that D.P. often cupped his hand over his right eye while reading. His mother had not noticed any "eye turns." D.P.'s history was otherwise unremarkable.

Clinical Findings		6 m	40 cm
Habitual Visual			
Acuity (VA):	OD	$20/30^{-2}$	20/20
	OS	20/200	20/20

Amplitude of Accommodation (w/o Rx): OD 10.00 diopters, OS 16.50 diopters

Retinoscopy:	OD	$-0.50 -0.25 \times 90$ $(20/20^{-1})$
	OS	-2.75 DS (20/20)
Subjective Refraction (SRx):	OD	-0.75 DS $(20/20^{+2})$
	OS	-2.75 DS $(20/20^{+2})$

Phorometry (w/SRx):	6 m	40 cm
Phoria	2^{Δ}XP	5^{Δ}XP'
Base-in (BI) vergence	X/14/8	20/25/16
Base-out (BO) vergence	19/28/12	16/24/12

Stereo Acuity (w/SRx): 20 seconds at 40 cm
Ocular Health: Normal

Trial Frame: D.P. felt comfortable at all viewing distances with the subjective refraction data.

Assessment
1. Simple myopia OU (OS > OD) and 2 diopters of anisometropia
2. Normal binocular vision

Treatment Plan
1. Rx: OD   −0.75 DS
       OS   −2.75 DS
2. Lens Design: Polycarbonate single vision lenses with standard (stock) base curves and center thicknesses. A standard design for each lens was used because no alteration in spectacle magnification was indicated.
3. Patient Education: D.P. was instructed to wear the glasses full time. He was cautioned that he might notice spatial distortion with the initial wearing of the prescription and that it would be important to wear the glasses constantly to accelerate adaptation. D.P. was instructed to return in 1 year for a follow-up examination.

Discussion
D.P. is the ideal patient for an optometrist's first encounter with anisometropia. It is worth one's time to think about why this case is "ideal" in order to prepare for more complicated cases of anisometropia. The following points highlight some of the clinical management issues that are discussed in detail later. Each of the three points should prompt consideration of other possibilities in other cases of anisometropia.

- Exact prescription and best visual acuity of each eye: With the spectacle prescription, D.P.'s vision was correctable to an acceptable and equal acuity in each eye.
- Binocularity: All the clinical findings, including the patient's positive response during trial framing, indicated that D.P. had good fusion with this prescription.
- Patient motivation to wear the prescription: D.P. presented with asthenopic symptoms, and it appeared the spectacle prescription would take care of the problem. D.P. noticed the improved, comfortable vision at all distances and did not feel the prescription made him "look funny."

The clinician often has to consider many factors before deciding a patient's final spectacle prescription. Certain types of cases cause the clinician to pause and think a bit longer than others. Prescribing for a patient with anisometropia is definitely one of those types.

Anisometropia (an/iso/metr/opia = without/equal/measurement/vision) is the condition in which the refractive error is different in the two eyes. Strictly speaking, nearly every patient has anisometropia because very few refractive errors are identical in each eye. Therefore the term *anisometropia* is usually reserved clinically for patients whose refractive error differs substantially between the two eyes. Low anisometropia is considered to be a difference of 2 diopters; high anisometropia is a difference greater than 2 diopters.[1]

Prescriptions for anisometropia vary from patient to patient by the dioptric difference between the two eyes, and they also vary by the nature of the ametropia itself. Every permutation exists. For example, one eye can be emmetropic and the other eye myopic, one eye can be emmetropic and the other hyperopic, one eye can be myopic and the other eye hyperopic (antimetropia), and so on. Anisometropia is not always a difference in spherical refractive error; it can be meridional, as in unilateral astigmatism.

The cases of anisometropia discussed in this chapter are cases of high anisometropia. The reason is simple. The vast majority of patients who have problems or potential problems with an anisometropic prescription are those with prescriptions in which the anisometropia is 2 diopters and greater.

Symptoms and Signs of Anisometropia

The clinical symptoms of anisometropia are highly variable. Symptoms are most often determined by both the type of anisometropia and how well the patient has adapted (or not adapted) to the anisometropic condition. For instance, patients with myopic anisometropia and patients with antimetropia often report monocular blur,[2] whereas patients with hyperopic anisometropia report headaches and asthenopia.[3] If the refractive difference between the two eyes is very large (>6 diopters), and if one eye is nearly emmetropic, the patient may not experience symptoms.[4] Other symptoms that may be reported with anisometropia include dizziness, diplopia, and nausea.[5]

Like the clinical symptoms associated with uncorrected anisometropia, the clinical signs also are varied. Among the possible manifestations are anisophoria, unequal accommodation, unequal aided or unaided acuities, tendency to close one eye, and strabismus. The universal sign of anisometropia is unequal refractive error between the two eyes.

Prescription Considerations and Guidelines

The ultimate goal in the treatment of patients with anisometropia is to provide a prescription that will result in good visual acuity in each eye and, despite the refractive difference, allow the patient to achieve comfortable binocular vision.

Determination of Refractive Error and Best Visual Acuity

First and foremost in the management of anisometropia is determination of the exact spectacle prescription and the best visual acuity in each eye. Without this information, the clinician is "flying blind" in an attempt to treat the patient.

Patients with anisometropia commonly have binocular problems associated with unilateral amblyopia or with a difference in perceived image size between the two eyes (that is, *aniseikonia*). As a result, standard refractive balance techniques that use patient comparisons of the two ocular images to balance the stimulus to accommodation often do not work. If the subjective refractive balance is suspect or impossible to determine, an accurate objective measurement must be made. This measurement can be taken by means of retinoscopy or autorefraction during cycloplegia.[6]

All patients need a properly balanced spectacle prescription; patients with anisometropia are no exception. If the prescription is not properly balanced, the patient can do nothing to provide simultaneous clear images in each eye. Because accommodation is consensual, a shift in accommodation to clear one eye simultaneously fogs the other eye by the same dioptric amount.

The adverse effects on central fusion caused by an improper refractive balance are well known. Some clinicians induce artificial anisometropia by means of unilateral fogging while they perform a refraction.[7] This technique produces central (foveal) suppression in the fogged eye and allows refraction of the unfogged eye while both eyes are open and maintaining peripheral fusion. The fact that this technique works effectively to disrupt central fusion speaks to the need for careful determination of the exact refractive error in a patient with anisometropia. Uncorrected anisometropia as small as 1 diopter can lead to amblyopia and poor binocular vision.[8] Normal fusion is not achieved in patients with anisometropia unless the correct refraction balance is in place.

In the clinical management of anisometropia, a prescription that incorporates the exact refractive balance is not always recommended. Patients with large amounts of anisometropia sometimes reject an initial prescription that incorporates the full balance found in a cycloplegic examination. Although the goal is to eventually prescribe the correct balance, some patients require progressive adaptation to this balance.

Amblyopia and Strabismus

The clinician should always carefully test for strabismus and amblyopia in patients with anisometropia. The fact that many patients with uncorrected anisometropia experience deprivational amblyopia that progresses to strabismus should be no surprise. If during the critical period of development, the retina does not receive a clear image, amblyopia develops. In addition, if one eye has a blurred retinal image and the other eye a clear retinal image, the development of sufficient binocular cortical neurons is prevented.[9] The abnormal development of the binocular visual system in many persons with uncorrected anisometropia helps explain why strabismus is not uncommon and why stereopsis with newly corrected anisometropia is often markedly decreased.

The presence of amblyopia and especially strabismus in patients with anisometropia necessitates that the clinician specifically address how these disorders will be treated. For example, a patient is not best served when a clinician conducts a careful refractive assessment, dispenses the appropriate spectacles, and then simply ignores that the patient is suppressing vision because of amblyopia or strabismus.

A full discussion of the methods of management of amblyopia and strabismus associated with anisometropia is beyond the scope of this chapter, but some important clinical guidelines are as follows:

1. The early diagnosis of anisometropia and treatment with an optical correction is essential if amblyopia is to be prevented.[10,11]
2. There are various methods of managing amblyopia, but the most common and basic approach to anisometropic amblyopia is provision of a clear retinal image through a full spectacle prescription followed by occlusion and binocular stimulus therapy.[12–15]
3. The success of strabismus vision therapy in a patient with anisometropia usually depends on the implementation and successful completion of amblyopia and binocular stimulus therapy.[12]
4. Age should not be a factor that automatically excludes a patient with anisometropic amblyopia from undergoing therapy. Therapy for anisometropic amblyopia has been demonstrated to be highly successful in both children and adults.[12,16–19]

Aniseikonia

Aniseikonia is the condition in which a patient perceives an image size difference between the two eyes. In a clinical setting, aniseikonia is most often considered (and therefore most often encountered) in the treatment of patients who present with large amounts of anisometropia. This is logical, but the clinician should always remember that symptoms resulting from aniseikonia are not exclusive to patients with anisometropia. Patients with nearly identical refractive errors (or those with equal retinal image sizes) may also perceive differences in image size between the two eyes.[20] Aniseikonia may therefore result from several sources, including differences in retinal image size commonly associated with anisometropia and differences in spatial density of the retinal photoreceptor elements.[21]

Aniseikonia research has a long and rich history.[22–24] Opinions regarding the clinical importance of aniseikonia and the appropriateness of regular testing and correction have been debated over the past several decades. Aniseikonia is now generally viewed as an important finding and is usually approached clinically when patients experience symptoms.

Several publications present in logical detail the clinical strategies and options for managing aniseikonia.[4,12,24–26] The following highlights some of the basic and most practical approaches and guidelines.

1. Be aware that aniseikonia may present in a patient with anisometropia and that aniseikonia may result when anisometropia is corrected with a refractive prescription.
2. Have a clinical method for detection and measurement of aniseikonia.
3. Develop a plan for the treatment of patients with aniseikonia and associated symptoms.

Anisometropia is generally classified as either refractive or axial in origin. In refractive anisometropia, the refractive surfaces of the optical components between the two eyes are different. In axial anisometropia, the axial lengths of the eyes are different. High anisometropia (>2 diopters) is typically, but not exclusively, axial in origin.[26]

Traditionally the clinical management of aniseikonia associated with anisometropia has been guided by Knapp's law. Knapp's law states that the retinal image size difference that results from axial anisometropia is minimized when the correcting spectacle lens is placed at the anterior focal plane of the eye.[4] When this law is applied, patients with axial anisometropia and aniseikonia are prescribed spectacles, and patients with refractive anisometropia and aniseikonia are prescribed contact lenses. Although the clinician should keep Knapp's law in mind in the management of aniseikonia, this conventional wisdom has been shown to have too many exceptions to remain a rigid clinical rule.[4,26] As a result, many clinicians try contact lenses as a first choice in the treatment of patients with anisometropia. This is not only preferable for cosmetic reasons but also often reduces or eliminates the aniseikonic symptoms.

The American Optical Office-Model Space Eikonometer (Buffalo, New York) has long been the instrument of choice for measuring aniseikonia.[24] It is no longer manufactured and is not readily available in optometric practices. As practical substitutes, several commercially manufactured tests now available allow measurement of aniseikonia.[12] Most of these tests have as their basis the simultaneous comparison of monocular images to determine if an image size difference exists.

If the clinician does not have an instrument to measure aniseikonia, all is not lost. The clinician can use several rules-of-thumb to help predict the amount of aniseikonia. There are several quick and easy tests to help estimate the amount of aniseikonia. The amount of anisometropia can be used as an estimate of the likely amount of aniseikonia. For every diopter of anisometropia, presume a 1% difference in the perceived image size between the two eyes.[25] Most patients can easily accept a 2% to 3% difference in retinal image size, but the clinician needs to remember that large individual variations in sensitivity exist.[4,24]

As a practical rule, the clinician should not be overly worried that aniseikonic symptoms will result in the rejection of an anisometropic prescription. Instead, the clinician should presume the patient will adapt.[27] The degree to which patients adapt to anisometropic prescriptions is very high, particularly among young patients. It is important to inform the patient that there will likely be a period of adaptation to the prescription and that wearing the prescription full time will accelerate adaptation. It is important to keep in mind that some patients may have persistent symptoms of aniseikonia and that the aniseikonia will have to be addressed.

A valuable clinical tool for management of aniseikonia is the iseikonic trial lens set.[28] These lenses (often referred to as "size" lenses) are manufactured to produce varying amounts of magnification (for example, 1 percent, 2 percent) and have no dioptric power. Placed over a patient's prescription, these lenses can be used to determine the amount of aniseikonia by means of equalization of the perceived image sizes between the two eyes. Iseikonic lenses are also helpful because they can be used as clip-on lenses to determine if a patient's symptoms are relieved by correction of the aniseikonia.[4]

When it has been determined that aniseikonia is causing symptoms in a patient with anisometropia and spectacles are to be prescribed, results with either the commercially available aniseikonia tests or the iseikonic trial lenses can be used to design a spectacle correction (or modify the existing spectacle correction) to reduce or eliminate the aniseikonia.[4,12,24,25,28]

Binocular Vision

Patients with anisometropia corrected with contact lenses have one notable advantage over their counterparts whose vision is corrected with spectacles. By the very nature of the spectacle anisometropic prescription, differential prismatic effects will be exerted on each eye as the eyes perform version and vergence movements. As long as the optical centers have been placed coincident with the pupillary centers in primary gaze, and the patient does not move his or her eyes, there will be no prismatic effect and therefore no problem. In reality, however, patients with spectacles do move their eyes.

Because the amount of spectacle prismatic effect can vary with direction of gaze, patients with spectacle-corrected anisometropia often demonstrate different amounts of heterophoria when tested in different directions of gaze. This is called *optical anisophoria.*[29,30] Optical anisophoria can produce the same asthenopic symptoms that occur with regular heterophorias and can lead to diplopia when the spectacle prism amount becomes too great and fusion is interrupted.

Optical anisophoria becomes a particular problem for patients with anisometropic presbyopia. When a bifocal lens is prescribed, the patient is forced to use a portion of the lens that is away from the distance optical center. If there is a substantial amount of anisometropia between the vertical meridians of the two eyes, a symptomatic induced vertical phoria may result.[31] The clinician should always examine the patient's spectacle prescription before prescribing a bifocal to determine if an induced vertical phoria is likely with down gaze. If it is, further testing through trial lenses is indicated before lenses are ordered. The symptoms caused by an induced vertical phoria in patients who are wearing bifocals for the first time are commonly not recognized by clinicians and are instead quickly attributed to an add power error.

Case Studies of Anisometropia

Patient P.P.

History: P.P., a 5-year-old girl, presented for her first eye examination. There were no reported vision problems from the patient or parents. The parents felt it was time for an examination. P.P.'s history was otherwise unremarkable.

Clinical Findings		6 m	40 cm
Habitual VA:	OD	20/200	20/200
	OS	20/30	20/40

Amplitude of Accommodation (w/o Rx): OD 6.25 diopters, OS 8.25 diopters

Retinoscopy:	OD	+4.00 −0.50 × 90 (20/200)
	OS	+2.00 DS (20/20^{-2})
SRx:	OD	+3.00 DS (20/200)
	OS	+1.00 DS (20/20^{-2})
Retinoscopy (w/ cycloplegia):	OD	+4.50 −0.50 × 80 (20/200)
	OS	+2.50 DS (20/20^{-2})

Phorometry (w/SRx): **6 m**   **40 cm**

   Phoria   1$^\Delta$EP   4$^\Delta$EP′

   BI vergence   No response because of suppression of OD

   BO vergence   No response because of suppression of OD

Ocular Health, Tonometry and Visual Fields: Normal OU

Assessment

1. Hyperopia OU (OD > OS), low astigmatism (against-the-rule), and 2 diopters of anisometropia
2. Refractive amblyopia OD
3. Intermittent suppression OD

Treatment Plan

1. Rx: OD   +3.50 –0.50 × 80

          OS   +1.50 DS

2. Lens Design: Polycarbonate single vision lenses with standard (stock) base curves and center thicknesses. A standard design for each lens was used because no alteration of spectacle magnification was indicated.
3. Vision therapy (occlusion therapy) for amblyopia OD
4. Patient Education: The patient was instructed to wear the glasses full-time. The need for a spectacle correction and for amblyopia therapy was explained to the parents.

Discussion

Compared with the case of D.P., this case is more typical of an anisometropic presentation. In particular, P.P. had hyperopic anisometropia with refractive amblyopia. As was the case with P.P., patients with anisometropia may not present with problems. Nor should the clinician depend too heavily on family members as a definitive guide for eliciting patient vision problems. Had someone simply occluded P.P.'s left eye, the initial negative reaction by the patient would have immediately been obvious and would have indicated a problem.

The management approach with P.P. was to maintain the refractive balance found with cycloplegic retinoscopy while moderately reducing symmetrically the amount of plus sphere for the first prescription. Prescribing the full amount of plus found during the cycloplegic examination is unwise. Nearly all patients reject such a prescription under noncyloplegic conditions because the prescription is overplussed at distance.[6]

If this patient is to regain binocularity, the amblyopia must be successfully treated. As the visual acuity of the right eye begins improving with the amblyopia therapy, antisuppression and binocular training will be needed to assure full binocular development.

Patient E.F.

History: E.F, a 2-year-old girl, presented with unilateral aphakia. A congenital cataract had been removed from the right eye 3 months prior. The patient had no optical or medical prescriptions and no other known ocular complications. Her history was otherwise unremarkable.

Clinical Findings

Retinoscopy: OD   +18.00 –0.50 × 180
                     OS   +1.00 DS

Retinoscopy (w/
  cycloplegia):   OD   +18.00 –0.50 × 180
                     OS   +2.00 –0.25 × 180

Cover Test and Hirschberg Test: No strabismus
Ocular Health: Normal OU other than aphakia OD

Assessment
1. Anisometropia secondary to unilateral aphakia OD
2. Binocularity is possible with correction of ametropia

Treatment Plan
1. Rx: OD   +20.00 D pediatric soft contact lens
        OS   no correction
2. Instructed the parents regarding contact lens application, removal, and cleaning
3. Monitored the contact lens fit and refractive error at regular 1-month follow-up visits
4. Provided vision therapy to prevent the development of refractive amblyopia
5. Parent Education: Explained that the optical correction OD and vision therapy are essential to prevent the development of refractive amblyopia

Discussion
E.F. had the extreme in acquired anisometropia. Because of her age, she was not an immediate candidate for an intraocular lens or refractive surgery, so a contact lens was essential if refractive amblyopia was to be prevented. The logic of the management was to prevent amblyopia and to provide regular follow-up examinations to monitor any changes in refractive error and binocular status. The contact lens power was overplussed to provide clear vision at near, since very young children engage in nearpoint activities much more than farpoint activities.

Patient R.D.

History: R.D., a 10-year-old boy, presented for his first eye examination. He reported that "I see blurry a lot and sometimes I see two." He also reported this had been occurring "for about a year." R.D.'s father commented that family members had noticed R.D. holding his reading material very close, and for the past year, they had noticed that R.D.'s left eye often turned out when he was reading. The history was otherwise unremarkable.

Clinical Findings		6 m	40 cm
Habitual VA:	OD	20/400	20/50
	OS	20/50	20/20

Amplitude of Accommodation (w/o Rx): OD 16.75 diopters, OS 11.00 diopters

Retinoscopy:	OD	−4.00 DS
	OS	−1.00 DS
SRx:	OD	−4.25 −0.25 × 60 (20/15^{-1})
	OS	−1.25 DS (20/15)

Phorometry (w/SRx):	6 m	40 cm
Phoria	2$^\Delta$XP	6$^\Delta$XP′
BI vergence	X/18/4	10/16/12
BO vergence	8/14/6	8/14/10

Stereo Acuity at 40 cm (w/SRx): 80 seconds
Aniseikonia Testing (w/SRx): 3 percent magnification OD needed for equal perceived image sizes
Stereo Acuity at 40 cm (w/Rx and 3 percent size lens OD): 60 seconds
Ocular Health: Normal OU
Trial Frame: R.D. stated that his vision was "more comfortable" at all viewing distances with a 3 percent size lens OD as compared with his vision without the size lens over the glasses.

Assessment

1. Simple myopia OU (OD > OS), low astigmatism (against-the-rule) OD, and 3 diopters of anisometropia
2. Aniseikonia of approximately 3 percent with prescription. Correction with a size lens OD yielded a small improvement in binocularity and notable decrease in asthenopia.
3. The parents' observation of intermittent left exotropia at near without the lenses was probably secondary to fusion loss associated with the uncorrected anisometropia.

Treatment Plan

1. Rx: OD   −4.25 −0.25 × 60 with 3 percent overall magnification
   OS   −1.25 DS
2. Lens Design: Because both lenses had a minus power, altering the lens design (that is, base curve and center thickness) provided only about 1.5 percent magnification OD. The OS base curve was flattened by 4 diopters relative to a standard corrective curve design combined with a decrease of the vertex distance OD by 3 mm relative to the OS. This was accomplished by appropriate positioning of the lens bevel. Polycarbonate single vision lenses were used.
3. Patient Education: R.D. was instructed to wear the glasses full time and to return 1 month after the lenses were dispensed for an assessment of binocular status. At the follow-up visit, the need for vision therapy to expand fusional ranges would be determined. The purpose of the spectacle correction with an image size adjustment was explained to the patient and his parents. R.D. was instructed to report any double vision or observable eye turns.

Discussion

The management approach with R.D. was the same as with the previous case studies except that in R.D.'s case a correction for aniseikonia was indicated to provide comfortable binocular vision. Because there was a history of an intermittent tropia, a follow-up examination to assess the patient's binocular status after wearing the prescription for 1 month was indicated.

Although specially designed spectacle lenses were prescribed for R.D., contact lenses should remain an option because the total spectacle magnification needed in the right eye was not achieved. The patient may experience asthenopia caused by the remaining uncorrected aniseikonia.

Patient S.S.

History: S.S., a 71-year-old woman, presented stating that "My eyes are too tired with my reading bifocals. I can't seem to get adjusted to read with them." She also reported that her vision at distance "has smoke over it." S.S. reported that these problems were of long standing. Her previous examination was 1 year prior. The ocular and medical histories were otherwise unremarkable for S.S.'s age.

Clinical Findings		6 m	40 cm
Habitual VA:	OD	20/25	20/25 with −2.50 −0.75 × 93
	OS	20/30	20/50 with +0.75 −2.00 × 88
			+2.00 D add OU

Cover test (w/HRx):		2^ΔXP	10^ΔXP'
Retinoscopy:	OD	$-2.00 -0.75 \times 120$	
	OS	$+1.75 -3.50 \times 90$	
SRx:	OD	$-2.25 -0.75 \times 90$ ($20/20^{-2}$)	
	OS	$+2.25 -3.50 \times 90$ ($20/20^{-2}$)	

Tentative Add at 40 cm: +2.50 D (20/20)

Phorometry (w/SRx):	6 m	40 cm (w/+2.50 D add)
Phoria	2^ΔXP	10^ΔXP'
BI vergence	X/12/8	X/22/16
BO vergence	X/12/4	X/6/0
Negative Relative Accommodation (NRA)/Positive Relative Accommodation (PRA)		+0.50/–0.25

Trial Frame: S.S. responded quite favorably to the subjective prescription for distance and a +2.50 D add for near.

Ocular Health, Tonometry and Visual Fields: Normal OU

Assessment

1. Antimetropia with compound myopic astigmatism OD and mixed astigmatism OS. Astigmatism is considerably higher OS
2. Anisometropia of 4.50 diopters in the 90° meridian and of 1.75 diopters in the 180° meridian
3. Normal binocularity with distance and near prescription in place
4. Moderate exophoria and low base-out vergence at near

Treatment Plan

1. Rx: OD $-2.25 -0.75 \times 90$ +2.50 D add
   OS $+2.25 -3.50 \times 90$ +2.50 D add
2. Lens Design: Hard resin (CR-39) multifocal lenses with FT 28 mm segments and duplication of the habitual base curves and center thicknesses because no alteration of these parameters was indicated
3. Patient Education: S.S. was advised about the change in her bifocal prescription. The prescription options for near were discussed. S.S. opted for a second pair of single vision spectacle lenses that contained her near prescription. She was also advised that she might notice spatial distortion the first time she wore both prescriptions. S.S. was instructed to drop her head while reading instead of dropping her eyes, as she was used to doing. S.S. understood that objects in the distance would be blurry while she wore the near prescription. S.S. was instructed to return in 1 year for a re-examination.

Discussion

S.S. had several problems that were solved with a new prescription. First, the distance prescription and add were not correct. With the new refractive results, the visual acuity improved as expected at far and near. Second, with the habitual prescription, S.S. was being forced to use the bifocal for near vision. Her distance prescription was causing a large amount of induced vertical prism, resulting in near-point asthenopia. To solve the vertical problem at near, the patient was given the option of a multifocal prescription with slab-off prism or two separate prescriptions. She chose the latter.

S.S. noticed the improvement with the new prescription and definitely wanted the change. Although the clinician should rightly be wary about altering an anisometropic prescription by a large amount in older patients, there are always exceptions. If the patient sees better with a new prescription, is motivated to use it, and understands the likely initial adaptation, then dispensing the prescription is the logical plan.

Patient A.P.

History: A.P., a 62-year-old man, presented for his annual eye examination. He stated that "I've been meaning to come in for a long time. I don't see very well far off with my right eye, and I don't need my bifocal anymore for my right eye. My left eye isn't bothering me." A.P. was in good health and was taking no medications. His history was otherwise unremarkable.

Clinical Findings		**6 m**	**40 cm**
Habitual VA:	OD	20/100	20/80 with −2.25 −0.50 × 80
	OS	20/20	20/20 with −0.75 −0.25 × 110
			+2.50 D add
Cover Test (w/HRx):		3^ΔXP	12^ΔXP′
Retinoscopy:	OD	−4.00 −0.25 × 90	
	OS	−2.00 DS	
SRx:	OD	−4.25 −0.25 × 85 (20/20^{-3})	
	OS	−2.00 −0.25 × 125 (20/20)	
Tentative Add at 40 cm:	+2.50 D (20/20)		

Phorometry (w/SRx):	**6 m**	**40 cm (w/+2.50 D add)**
Phoria	3^ΔXP	12^ΔXP′
BI vergence	X/14/6	X/20/18
BO vergence	X/12/4	X/8/2
NRA/PRA		+0.25/−0.50

Trial Frame: A.P. felt he saw well with the subjective refraction data and a +2.50 D add, but he did notice that the walls were "a bit slanted." He stated he wanted the new prescription. Nearpoint vertical phoria testing indicated that A.P. would have normal vertical fusion when lowering his eyes to view through the bifocal segment.

Aniseikonia Testing: 2% magnification OD required for equal perceived image sizes. Placement of a 2% size lens over the right eye in a trial frame produced no noticeable difference to A.P. in terms of visual acuity or vision comfort.

Ocular Health, Tonometry and Visual Fields: Normal except for lenticular nuclear sclerosis and incipient cataract OD

Assessment
1. Acquired myopic anisometropia (OD > OS) secondary to lenticular index changes due to nuclear sclerosis OD
2. Very slight decrease of best visual acuity OD secondary to cataract
3. Aniseikonia (2%) secondary to acquired anisometropia. Ocular image OS is larger than OD.

Treatment Plan
1. Rx: OD $-4.25 -0.25 \times 85 + 2.50$ D add
       OS $-2.00 -0.25 \times 125 + 2.50$ D add
2. Lens Design: Hard resin (CR-39) multifocal lenses with FT-25 mm segments and a duplication of his habitual base curves and center thicknesses because no alteration of these parameters was indicated.
3. Patient Education: The lenticular changes OD and how the cataract had changed the prescription were explained to A.P. The initial spatial distortion that occurs with a new prescription of this kind and the adaptation that would take place if the prescription were worn full-time were discussed. A.P. was instructed to return in 1 year for a re-examination.

Discussion
Acquired anisometropia secondary to lenticular changes is not uncommon. Both the best corrected visual acuity and the minimal induced aniseikonia allowed this patient to continue functioning with a new prescription.

The surgical alteration of refractive error is now common. Most often when surgical intervention is performed to reduce ametropia, the surgeon attempts to take each eye to emmetropia in sequential operations. If treatment is successful, there will be no clinically significant anisometropia.

With unilateral cataract extraction and intraocular lens implant, patients are often left with the pseudophakic eye near emmetropia and the other eye at the unaltered level of ametropia. Fortunately, many patients adapt to this type of acquired anisometropia, but the clinician must be aware that some do not.[32,33] The clinician must also be aware of the possibility of symptoms of acquired anisometropia and aniseikonia in any patient who has undergone an ocular surgery (unilateral or bilateral) in which the refractive error has been altered.

Although the foregoing discussion of acquired anisometropia is restricted to refractive anisometropia, the clinician should remember that acquired anisometropia can also be axial in origin. Some examples of acquired axial anisometropia and their causes include scleral buckle operations, retrobulbar mass, central serous retinopathy, and asymmetric (unilateral) posterior pole staphyloma progression in pathologic myopia. During an eye examination, the clinician should always determine the origin of acquired anisometropia.

Patient S.K.

History: S.K., a 28-year-old woman, had not undergone an eye examination in 10 years. She also never had a prescription. Her symptoms related to difficulty driving at night. She reported that "I see starbursts at night while I'm driving. Cars approaching me look like they are going to hit me." Her history was otherwise unremarkable.

Clinical Findings		6 m	40 cm
Habitual VA:	OD	20/25^{+1}	20/20^{-1}
	OS	20/200	20/20

Amplitude of Accommodation (w/o Rx): OD 5.25 diopters, OS 9.00 diopters

Retinoscopy:	OD	$+0.25 -1.00 \times 175$ (20/15$^{-2)}$
	OS	$-1.50 -1.00 \times 180$ (20/25^{-1})
SRx:	OD	$+0.25 -0.50 \times 178$ (20/15^{-1})
	OS	$-2.25 -0.50 \times 160$ (20/15^{-2})

Phorometry (w/SRx):	6 m	40 cm
Phoria	3$^{\Delta}$XP	4$^{\Delta}$XP'
BI vergence	X/10/4	10/18/8
BO vergence	16/20/12	22/28/18

Stereo Acuity at 40 cm (w/SRx): 60 seconds

Trial Frame: S.K. noticed her vision was "somewhat better" with the subjective refraction, but flatly stated, "I don't want to wear glasses."

Assessment
1. Antimetropia with mixed astigmatism OD and compound myopic astigmatism OS
2. Anisometropia (2.50 diopters)
3. Stereo acuity mildly reduced at near

Treatment Plan

1. Rx: Because S.K. refused correction with spectacle lenses, she was scheduled for a contact lens fitting.
2. Patient Education: The nature of S.K.'s refractive errors and the necessity for a full-time prescription for clear, comfortable vision at all viewing distances were explained. She was instructed to return for a contact lens fitting.

Discussion

This patient is a "natural monofit," meaning that without any correction she sees well at distance with her right eye and that at near she sees well with her left eye. These patients are commonly content to leave their vision uncorrected. When prescribing for this kind of anisometropia, the clinician should take the time to carefully explain to the patient the benefits of the prescription. Otherwise the patient is likely to not wear the prescription long enough to adapt.

Summary

As a practical summary to the treatment of patients with anisometropia, the clinician should keep the following points in mind.

- Determine the precise refractive error.
- Determine the patient's binocular status with and without the prescription. Accurately assess any amblyopia and strabismus.
- Be prepared to assess and treat aniseikonia.
- Develop a treatment plan that has clear objectives, including expectations of the patient's binocular status.
- Ensure that the treatment plan matches the patient's needs.
- Take the extra time to explain to the patient the nature of the refractive error and what the treatment plan is going to do.

References

1. Borish IM. *Clinical Refraction.* 2nd ed. Chicago: Professional Press, 1970:257–304.
2. Goss DA. *Ocular Accommodation, Convergence, and Fixation Disparity.* Boston: Butterworth-Heinemann, 1986:149.
3. Milder B, Rubin ML. *The Fine Art of Prescribing Glasses Without Making a Spectacle of Yourself.* 2nd ed. Gainesville, Fla: Triad, 1991:179–218.
4. Bartlett JD. Anisometropia and aniseikonia. In: Amos JF, ed. *Diagnosis and Management in Vision Care.* Boston: Butterworth-Heinemann, 1987:173–202.

5. McKee MC, Provines WF. Nausea caused by aniseikonia. *Am J Optom Physiol Opt* 1987;64:221–223.

6. Amos JF. Cycloplegic refraction. In: Bartlett JD, Jannus SD, eds. *Clinical Ocular Pharmacology.* Boston: Butterworth-Heinemann, 1989:421–429.

7. Humphriss D. Binocular refraction. In: Edwards K, Llewellyn R, eds. *Optometry.* London: Butterworth-Heinemann, 1988:140–149.

8. Ingram RM, Walker C. Refraction as a means of predicting squint or amblyopia in preschool siblings of children known to have these defects. *Br J Ophthalmol* 1979;63:238–242.

9. Schwartz SH. *Visual Perception: A Clinical Orientation.* Norwalk, Conn: Appleton & Lange, 1994:324–325.

10. Tanlamai T, Goss DA. Prevalence of monocular amblyopia among anisometropes. *Am J Optom Physiol Opt* 1979;56:704–715.

11. Amos JF. Refractive amblyopia: a preventable vision condition. *J Am Optom Assoc* 1979;50:1153–1159.

12. Scheiman M, Wick B. *Clinical Management of Binocular Vision.* Philadelphia: Lippincott, 1994:490–508.

13. Griffin JR. *Binocular Anomalies: Procedures for Vision Therapy.* 2nd ed. Chicago: Professional Press, 1982:75–76,195–196.

14. Press LJ. Amblyopia. *J Optom Vision Dev* 1988;19:2–15.

15. Sherman A. Alternative treatment for anisometropic amblyopic patients: a case report. *J Optom Vision Dev* 1993;24:25–28.

16. Kivlin JD, Flynn JT. Therapy of anisometropic amblyopia. *J Pediatr Ophthalmol Strab* 1981;18:47–56.

17. Lithander J, Sjostrand J. Anisometropia and strabismic amblyopia in the age group 2 years and above: a prospective study of the results of treatment. *Br J Ophthalmol* 1991;75:111–116.

18. Kutschke PJ, Scott WE, Keech RV. Anisometropic amblyopia. *Ophthalmology* 1991;98:258–263.

19. Wick B, Wingard M, Cotter S, Scheiman M. Anisometropic amblyopia: is the patient ever too old to treat? *Optom Vision Sci* 1992;69:866–878.

20. Rabin J, Bradley A, Freeman RD. On the relationship between aniseikonia and axial anisometropia. *Am J Optom Physiol Opt* 1983;60:553–558.

21. Bradley A, Rabin J, Freeman RD. Non optical determinants of aniseikonia. *Ophthalmol Vision Sci* 1983;24:507–512.

22. Bannon RE. Developments in the field of aniseikonia. In: *Transactions of the International Optical Congress.* London: British Optical Association, 1951:151–164.

23. Bannon RE. Clinical Manual on Aniseikonia. Buffalo: *American Optical,* 1976:4–13.

24. Bannon RE. Aniseikonia. In: Duane TD, ed. *Clinical Ophthalmology.* Hagerstown, Md: Harper & Row, 1979;1–5.

25. Fannin TE, Grosvenor T. *Clinical Optics.* Boston: Butterworth-Heinemann, 1987:321–358.

26. Laird IK. Anisometropia. In: Grosvenor T, Flom MC, eds. *Refractive Anomalies.* Boston: Butterworth-Heinemann, 1991;174–198.

27. Carter DB. Symposium on conventional wisdom in optometry. *Am J Optom Arch Am Acad Optom* 1967;44:731–745.

28. Kleinstein RN. Iseikonic trial lenses: an aid in diagnosing aniseikonia. *Optom Monthly* 1978;69:132–137.

29. Cline D, Hofstetter HW, Griffin JR. *Dictionary of Visual Science.* 4th ed. Radnor, Pa: Chilton, 1989:37.

30. Garcia G, Pavan-Langston D. Refractive errors and clinical optics. In: Pavan-Langston D, ed. *Manual of Ocular Diagnosis and Therapy.* Boston: Little, Brown, 1991:361–388.

31. Amos JF. Induced hyperphoria in anisometropic presbyopia. *J Am Optom Assoc* 1991;62:664–671.

32. Katsumi O, Miyajima H, Ogawa T, Hirose T. Aniseikonia and stereoacuity in pseudophakic patients. *Ophthalmology* 1992;99:1270–1277.

33. Enoch JM. Aniseikonia and intraocular lenses: a continuing saga. *Optom Vision Sci* 1994;71:67–68.

Case Study Exercises

For each case study, determine the diagnosis and develop a treatment plan. The clinical questions provided with each case may assist you by highlighting important aspects of the case.

Patient L.L.

History: L.L., a 7-year-old boy, presents for his first eye examination. He states that "I can't see the blackboard at school." He has no other symptoms. The history is otherwise unremarkable.

Clinical Findings		6 m	40 cm
Habitual VA:	OD	20/40^{+2}	20/20
	OS	20/200	20/200

Amplitude of Accommodation (w/o Rx): OD 12.00 diopters, OS 15.75 diopters

Retinoscopy:	OD	$-1.00 -0.25 \times 180$
	OS	$-3.00 -0.25 \times 10$
SRx:	OD	$-0.75 -0.25 \times 180$ (20/20$^{+1)}$)
	OS	$-3.00 -0.25 \times 10$ (20/20^{+2})

Phorometry (w/SRx):	6 m	40 cm
Phoria	2$^\Delta$XP	4$^\Delta$XP'
BI vergence	X/16/8	22/25/16
BO vergence	20/28/14	18/24/12

Stereo Acuity at 40 cm (w/SRx): 40 seconds

Clinical Questions
1. What would you prescribe for this patient?
2. What level of binocularity do you expect this person to have?
3. When would you examine this patient again?

Patient D.T.

History: D.T., a 6-year-old boy, presents for his first eye examination. The patient and parents report no visual problems at home or at school. The history is unremarkable.

Clinical Findings		6 m	40 cm
Habitual VA:	OD	20/400	20/400
	OS	20/30	20/40
Cover Test (w/o Rx):		5$^\Delta$RET	10$^\Delta$RET'

Amplitude of Accommodation: OD no response, OS 8.25 diopters

Retinoscopy:	OD	+5.00 –0.50 × 90 (20/400)
	OS	+1.00 DS (20/20^{-2})
SRx:	OD	+5.00 DS (20/400 w/poor response)
	OS	+0.50 DS (20/20)
Retinoscopy (w/cycloplegia):	OD	+6.25 –0.50 × 80 (20/400)
	OS	+2.25 DS (20/20^{-4})

| Cover Test (w/cycloplegia): | 6 m | 40 cm |
| | No tropia | 4$^\Delta$RET |

Ocular Health: Normal OU

Clinical Questions
1. What would you prescribe for this patient?
2. Is aniseikonia a concern in this case when the patient begins wearing a spectacle prescription? How might the aniseikonia be minimized?
3. What treatment strategy might assist this patient's binocularity?

Patient A.T.

History: A.T., a 70-year-old woman, presents with a concern about her left eye. She states that, "My left eye isn't as good as my right eye." She also reports that she has noticed this for "many months," and it has gradually become worse. A.T.'s ocular and medical history are unremarkable for her age. Her last eye examination was 2 years prior.

Clinical Findings		**6 m**	**40 cm**
Habitual VA:	OD	20/25	20/25 with plano –0.50 × 180
	OS	20/100	20/100 with +0.75 –0.25 × 175
			+2.50 D add OU
Cover Test (w/HRx):		4$^\Delta$XP	10$^\Delta$XP′_
Retinoscopy:	OD	–0.25 –0.50 × 180	
	OS	–2.25 –1.50 × 180	
SRx:	OD	–0.25 –0.25 × 180 (20/25^{+3})	
	OS	–2.50 –1.25 × 180 (20/25^{-1})	

Tentative Add at 40 cm: +2.50 D (20/25)

Phorometry (w/SRx):	**6 m**	**40 cm (w/+2.50 D add)**
Phoria	3$^\Delta$XP	10$^\Delta$XP′
BI vergence	X/16/8	X/18/16
BO vergence	X/10/2	X/7/2
NRA/PRA		+0.25/–0.25

Trial Frame: A.T. feels she sees very clearly at distance with the new spectacle prescription, but she reports that she feels nauseated when she looks around the examination room. While the clinician is determining an add power in the trial frame, A.T. states it "feels like her eyes are pulling apart" when she drops her eyes to read.

Ocular Health, Tonometry and Visual Fields: Normal for the patient's age OU

Clinical Questions
1. Why does the patient feel nauseated during trial framing of the subjective refraction data?
2. Why does it feel like the patient's eyes are pulling apart when she drops her eyes to read?
3. What other tests should be conducted if any?
4. What would you prescribe for this patient?

Patient F.F.

History: F.F., a 12-year-old boy, presents wearing a spectacle prescription and reports he has undergone numerous eye examinations since he was 4 years of age. His mother mentions that one eye doctor years prior talked about patching and vision therapy, but none was ever done. F.F.'s only symptom is occasional blur while reading. His history is otherwise unremarkable.

Clinical Findings		6 m	40 cm
Habitual VA:	OD	$20/20^{-2}$	20/20 with +4.00 DS
	OS	20/20	20/20 with +2.00 DS

Amplitude of Accommodation (w/HRx): OD 6.75 diopters, OS 8.25 diopters

Cover Test (w/HRx): The unilateral cover test shows no tropia at 6 m or 40 cm. The alternating cover test shows a "unilateral" left esophoria at distance.

Retinoscopy:	OD	$+5.00 -0.50 \times 180$ (20/20)
	OS	+2.25 DS (20/20)
SRx:	OD	$+4.25 -0.50 \times 180$ (20/20)
	OS	+2.00 DS (20/20)

Phorometry (w/SRx):	6 m	40 cm
Phoria	ortho	$3^{\Delta}EP'$
BI vergence	X/12/6	12/18/8
BO vergence	22/28/16	30/34/24

Stereo Acuity at 40 cm (w/SRx): 60 seconds

Retinoscopy (w/ cycloplegia):	OD	$+6.00 -0.50 \times 180$
	OS	+2.75 DS

Ocular Health, Tonometry and Visual Fields: Normal OU

Clinical Questions

1. What condition or conditions would cause a unilateral phoria?
2. What is likely the cause of the blur at near?
3. Would a full plus prescription (that is, cycloplegic refraction data) be appropriate for this patient? If not, how would you modify the prescription?

6   Low Ametropias

Kenneth E. Brookman

A Case Study of Low Ametropia

History: C.J., a 22-year-old student, presented with symptoms of "tired eyes" and "sleepiness" after studying for about 60 to 90 minutes. He reported that his vision at distance and near seemed fine most of the time but that distance vision appeared a little blurred when his eyes felt tired. He had no previous prescription. The personal and family histories were unremarkable.

Clinical Findings		6 m	40 cm
Habitual Visual			
Acuity (VA):	OD	20/20^{+2}	20/20
	OS	20/20	20/20
Cover Test (w/o Rx):		ortho	ortho'
Near Point of Convergence (NPC): 3 cm			
Stereo Acuity at 40 cm (w/o Rx): 30 seconds (Randot)			
Retinoscopy:	OD	+0.25 DS	
	OS	+0.50 –0.25 × 180	
Subjective Refrac-			
tion (SRx):	OD	+0.25 –0.25 × 175 (20/15^{-2})	
	OS	+0.50 –0.50 × 180 (20/15^{-1})	

Phorometry (w/Rx):	6 m	40 cm
Phoria	ortho	3$^{\Delta}$XP'
Base-in (BI) vergence	X/8/5	12/22/15
Base-out (BO) vergence	X/12/8	14/25/20
Amplitude of Accommodation: >8.00 diopters OD, OS, OU		

Ocular Health, Tonometry and Visual Fields: Normal
Trial Frame: C.J. preferred the subjective refraction data and reported clear and comfortable vision.

Assessment
1. Symptoms of tired eyes, a feeling of sleepiness, and transient blurred vision at distance associated with reading for a relatively short period of time most likely resulting from low ametropia of each eye, and possibly also due to the very slight amsometropia.
2. Very low simple hyperopic astigmatism of both eyes, the astigmatism in the left eye being slightly greater than that in the right
3. Binocular vision functions (phorias, vergences, and accommodation) normal for the patient's age

Treatment Plan
1. Rx: OD   +0.25 –0.25 × 175
       OS   +0.50 –0.50 × 180
2. Lens Design: Single vision untinted resin (CR-39) lenses
3. Patient Education: C.J. was instructed to wear the lenses during all nearpoint tasks, and for distance tasks as needed to improve visual acuity and enhance vision comfort. A re-examination in 1 year was recommended.

Discussion
This case study is quite typical of the clinical presentation of patients with low ametropia. Symptoms are often mild and sometimes vague and usually are manifested during a detailed vision task, such as reading.[1] The symptoms presented by C.J. were not specifically diagnostic of low ametropia, since they also could be associated with other vision anomalies, such as those related to deficiencies of the vergence and accommodation systems. However, in the absence of test results that indicate such deficiencies (that is, all binocular vision functions were normal for C.J.'s age), and considering the refractive findings and uncorrected visual acuity, the diagnostic association between the patient's symptoms and the uncorrected low ametropia is the most justifiable. Correction of this type of ametropia with spectacle lenses, whether it be myopia, hyperopia, or astigmatism, often results in immediate comfort for the patient. Therefore, the prognosis in these types of cases is generally very good.

Symptoms and Signs of Low Ametropia

Patients with low ametropia (that is, myopia, hyperopia, and astigmatism of less than 1 diopter) often pose a unique management challenge. This is especially true of patients with low hyperopia and astigmatism. For these patients, symptoms resulting from uncorrected ametropia are often vague, transient, and difficult to articulate. Clinical findings for these patients are usually normal or very near normal, and therefore may seem clinically insignificant.

Of the three most common symptoms associated with uncorrected or undercorrected ametropia, that is, blurred vision, asthenopia (which could be reported as eye strain, fatigue, or discomfort), and asthenopic headache, any or all of them may be reported by a patient with a low ametropia. Often blurred vision resulting from low ametropia is very subtle and has little if any effect on visual acuity since the defocusing of the retinal image is minimal. In the case of hyperopia and astigmatism, accommodation may compensate for the refractive error. Even so, the effects may still be manifested or intensified as asthenopia or a headache when associated with an intense or detailed vision task, such as occupational or recreational reading and the use of video display terminals (VDTs). These symptoms may arise from fatigue of the ciliary system because of the prolonged near work combined with a " . . . slight overexertion of accommodation."[1]

Many investigators have shown an association between the use of VDTs and vision-related symptoms, including headache, slowness in refocusing between near and distant objects, double vision, blurred vision, eye irritation, and eye strain.[2-6] The etiology of these symptoms is often unclear, because environmental factors (for example, the type of visual task, work pressure, work interest, and frequency of breaks) and ocular factors (for example, refractive error, accommodation amplitude, heterophoria, and vergence range) have been identified as potential causes.[2-6]

Daum et al. suggested an association between low uncorrected ametropia in particular with symptoms from VDT use, such as slow refocusing from near to distance objects, especially with low myopia and astigmatism, and eyestrain.[2] They commented that correcting these low ametropias is a factor in minimizing the symptoms. In addition, they suggested that other potential contributing factors need to be considered before one prescribes lenses to VDT users.

Low myopia usually is manifested as a reduction in visual acuity and therefore is often easier to diagnose than hyperopia or astigmatism. Headaches due to excessive squinting to clear distance vision may also arise in patients with myopia or myopic astigmatism.[1] Symptoms that seem unrelated to the eyes, such as general body fatigue, may also occur as a result of uncorrected low ametropia.[7]

The predominant clinical signs for the diagnosis of low ametropias are the objective and subjective refraction data. Certain low ametropias (that is, hyperopia and astigmatism), however, may be difficult to neutralize with corrective lenses. With these ametropias, visual acuity often changes little with the addition of lenses because of compensation by accommodation, and patient responses during a subjective refraction can be uncertain or variable. Low myopia, on the other hand, is perhaps the easiest condition to identify during a refraction, because its correction usually results in improvement in visual acuity. Nevertheless, "a precise and careful subjective refraction " is essential to diagnosis and management of these conditions regardless of the ametropia.[1]

Case studies reported as early as the late 19th century by Hamilton and by White showed a strong association between symptoms of asthenopia and uncorrected low astigmatism.[8,9] Whether this association represents a cause-and-effect relation may be debatable, although even today patients with low ametropia quite often report symptoms of asthenopia. On the basis of their observations, Hamilton and White agreed that a very low cylinder lens (that is, 0.25 diopter) has some value in relieving symptoms of asthenopia. Cholerton, however, suggested that a low cylinder prescription may have only a placebo effect, especially in the absence of a noticeable improvement in visual acuity.[10]

The case history of a patient with low ametropia is particularly important for the diagnosis and treatment plan. The clinician must identify symptoms and their association with specific vision tasks and determine the environment in which the tasks are performed.[1]

The clinician must also explore any patient anxiety or concern about the symptoms. Nathan suggested that patients with symptoms of "eyestrain" often have an "ocular fear" of a more serious vision problem.[11] The case history can be quite useful in assessing this fear and reassuring the patient.

Blume referred to anecdotal evidence that suggested an association between certain personality types and low ametropia accompanied by symptoms of asthenopia.[1] That is, a patient's response to uncorrected low ametropia may be due in part to his or her personality characteristics. For example, patients who are detail-oriented, precise, and intense may experience symptoms of these ametropias more often than patients who do not have these characteristics. Nevertheless, the symptoms are real and may certainly compromise vision efficiency and comfort regardless of the patient's personality.

Prescription Considerations and Guidelines

Symptoms of blurred vision, asthenopia, and headache resulting from uncorrected low ametropia can affect patients of all ages. Since symptoms most often originate with detailed vision tasks, especially at near, patients who do not engage in these types of tasks, such as young children, usually have no symptoms. An older child or an adult may report any or all of these symptoms depending on the type and severity of the ametropia and the nature of their vision tasks.

The management strategy for low ametropia depends on a number of factors, including the presence and severity of symptoms and the effect of the ametropia on visual acuity. In some cases of low ametropia, such as simple hyperopia of a young patient with a normal amplitude of accommodation, symptoms usually are minimal if present at all, and visual acuity at distance and near is likely to be normal. In these cases, no corrective lenses for distance or near are indicated. The patients should be educated, however, about the nature of their condition and the symptoms and signs. Reassuring patients that the condition will not lead to vision loss or other serious complications is important.

The prevailing clinical question that must be addressed in the management of a low ametropia is "To prescribe or not to prescribe?" For patients of almost any age who have symptoms, there is a strong association between the symptoms and low ametropia whether myopia, hyperopia, or astigmatism. The most appropriate management strategy in these cases is to prescribe corrective lenses to fully neutralize the ametropia.

Because the magnitude of the corrective lens powers is small for these patients, modification of the prescription to enhance adaptation to the lenses or to prevent secondary symptoms, such as those from the effect of the prescription on binocular vision or accommodation, is not usually a consideration. However, the patient may be instructed to wear the lenses at certain times or at certain viewing distances to maintain vision efficiency and comfort. For example, a patient with low myopia who shows an esophoria at near through the distance prescription may be instructed to remove the lenses for all near work to reduce the esophoria and maintain normal binocular function. As a general guideline, however, patients should use their lenses for the greatest benefit, which may be full-time wear.

When low ametropia is corrected, patients with symptoms often report almost immediate relief, especially if the symptoms arise during a specific vision task. These patients usually adapt quite easily to their prescription whether they are first-time or habitual lens wearers. Blume reported on a number of these types of cases.[1]

The relative certainty or uncertainty of patient responses during a subjective refraction can often assist the clinician in management decisions by allowing determination of the clinical significance of low ametropia and its correction. It also allows the clinician to assess the likelihood that a patient will benefit from corrective lenses. That is, the more certain the patient responses, the greater likelihood that there will be a benefit.

Demonstration of the benefits of corrective lenses may be easily accomplished with the use of trial lenses and a trial frame. The patient may observe immediate improvement in visual acuity with certain ametropias, and, perhaps more important, feel improved vision comfort and absence of asthenopia or headache when performing a vision task such as reading or VDT use. A demonstration of improved vision comfort, however, is unlikely to occur immediately. These demonstrations also serve to enhance patient confidence in the treatment plan and in the clinician.

The prognosis in any case becomes quite good when the patient has confidence in the treatment plan. This confidence is often instilled when the benefits of the treatment are made apparent to the patient, as with trial lens demonstration and patient education.

Accommodation and Vergence

The prescription of spherical and cylindrical spectacle lenses to manage any ametropia has the potential to affect the accommodation and vergence systems to a point where dysfunction may occur. Plus and minus lenses, whether spherical or cylindrical, alter the stimulus to the accommodation system and thus may alter the patient's accommodation response. In addition, as accommodation is affected, so is the vergence system, because of the close relation between these two functions. As accommodation increases from a habitual state, so does convergence. This could yield a possible overconvergence, which would place a greater demand on fusional divergence. Conversely, underconvergence due to a decrease of accommodation from a habitual state would place a greater demand on fusional convergence. Greater demands on these functions might certainly result in associated symptoms such as asthenopia and headache.

The prismatic effect from spectacle lenses when an individual moves his or her eyes from side to side or up and down might also affect vergence and accommodation. The magnitudes of these effects, however, are likely a function of the magnitude of the lens powers. In any case, it is important that the clinician consider these potential effects before prescribing lenses.

With low-power spectacle lenses, a clinically significant effect on the accommodation and vergence systems is not expected. In fact, patients who experience symptoms of asthenopia or asthenopic headache from an uncorrected low ametropia, often report immediate relief of these symptoms with a refractive correction. Nevertheless, patients who are prescribed low-power lenses need to be educated about spectacle lens adaptations and monitored for symptoms related to accommodation or vergence dysfunction.

Spectacle Design

The design of low-power spectacle lenses is usually quite straightforward. Lens design features such as base curves and center thickness are fairly standard and readily available as stock lenses. Little if any special design considerations are required except perhaps with respect to occupational multifocal lenses. In these cases, consideration must be given to factors such as the patients' working distances, the level of the vision task (that is, above, below, or at eye level), and illumination in the workplace. There are usually little to no restrictions with regard to frame size or frame design for use with low-power lenses.

Case Studies of Low Ametropia

Patient R.B.

History: R.B., a 10-year-old boy presented with a symptom blurred vision at distance. He noticed his vision was blurred when he viewed the chalkboard in school. R.B. was not bothered by the blurred vision at any other time. He did report that he sat toward the back of the classroom. R.B. commented that moving toward the front of the room helped quite a bit. He expressed no problems when reading. R.B.'s various activities outside school were fairly typical for a boy his age. R.B. had undergone no previous eye examinations. His personal and family histories were unremarkable.

Clinical Findings		**6 m**	**40 cm**
Habitual VA:	OD	$20/20^{-3}$	20/20
	OS	$20/25^{-1}$	20/20
Cover Test (w/o Rx):		ortho	ortho'
NPC: 2 cm			
Stereo Acuity at 40 cm (w/o Rx): 40 seconds (Randot)			
Keratometry:	OD	44.00/43.50 at 180° (with-the-rule)	
	OS	44.00/43.50 at 180° (with-the-rule)	
Retinoscopy:	OD	$-0.25 -0.25 \times 180$	
	OS	-0.25 DS	
SRx:	OD	-0.25 DS $(20/20^{+2})$	
	OS	-0.50 DS $(20/20^{+3})$	

Phorometry (w/Rx):	**6 m**	**40 cm**
Phoria	2^{Δ}EP	6^{Δ}EP'
BI vergence	X/12/6	X/16/8
BO vergence	X/24/12	X/24/10

Amplitude of Accommodation: >10.00 diopters OD, OS, OU

Trial Frame: R.B. noticed immediate improvement in his acuity and did not desire any modification from the subjective refraction data.

Assessment

1. Reduced visual acuity at distance due to low amount of simple myopia of both eyes, myopia in the left eye being slightly greater
2. Slight over convergence at distance and near viewing through the prescription with adequate compensating (BI) vergences at both distances

Treatment Plan

1. Option 1: Rx: OD –0.25 DS
                        OS –0.50 DS

   Option 2: No Rx
2. Lens Design: Polycarbonate single vision lenses in a sturdy frame
3. Patient Education: The parents and patient were presented with two options. If option 1 were selected, R.B. would use the glasses primarily in the classroom for distance viewing but would remove them for sustained near work. He could then remain seated at his present location in the classroom. If option 2 were selected, R.B. would most likely have to move to the front of the classroom for viewing the chalkboard. The parents were reassured that if no lenses were prescribed, R.B.'s myopia would neither necessarily worsen nor improve.

Discussion

This case illustrates the importance of the case history in determining the treatment options for low ametropia and presenting these options to the patient and parents. R.B.'s history showed rather infrequent reports of mild blurred vision at distance, which suggests that he was bothered very little by this blurred vision. In addition, R.B.'s slightly reduced visual acuity seemed to have little effect on his achievement in school and during other activities. In fact, at near the uncorrected myopia (which is equivalent to adding plus) proved to be a slight advantage for R.B., because it helped to reduce his overconvergence by reducing the stimulus to accommodation.

With consideration to R.B.'s history and his vision function without a refractive correction, the option of no prescription was certainly viable. Because the responsibility of an optometrist, as well as that of any health care practitioner, is to present the viable treatment options to patients and assist them in their decision, the options of prescription and no prescription were presented here. A complete discussion of the advantages and disadvantages of both options, including a prognosis, is essential. In this case the parents elected to wait on the prescription and have R.B. re-examined in 1 year, or sooner if symptoms worsened.

In cases of an early-developing ametropia, especially myopia, the parents need to understand the potential time course of the condition.

They also need to understand that receiving a prescription now or waiting will neither worsen nor improve the condition in any predictable way. Heredity, of course, is a factor in developing ametropia, especially myopia, and therefore needs to be explored in the history.

Patient J.M.

History: J.M., a 47-year-old woman, presented with a desire to update her current single vision prescription for near only. Her habitual prescription (HRx) was 2 years old. She felt that her reading vision had decreased slightly during the past year. In particular, J.M. noticed slight blurring of telephone directory print and difficulty threading a needle with her glasses on. Distance vision presented no problem for her. J.M. was in good health, although she had borderline hypertension. Her blood pressure was being monitored periodically. She was taking no medications. J.M.'s other personal and family histories were unremarkable.

Clinical Findings		**6 m**	**40 cm**
Uncorrected VA:	OD	$20/20^{-3}$	$20/40^{-2}$
	OS	$20/20^{-2}$	20/40
Habitual VA:	OD		$20/30^{-2}$ with +1.00 DS
	OS		$20/25^{-1}$ with +1.00 DS
Cover Test (w/HRx):		ortho	ortho'

NPC: 3 cm

Stereo Acuity at 40 cm (w/HRx): 20 seconds (Randot)

Keratometry:	OD	43.75/43.25 at 90° (against-the-rule)
	OS	44.00/43.75 at 90° (against-the-rule)
Retinoscopy:	OD	+0.75 –0.25 ×85
	OS	+0.50 –0.25 × 80
SRx:	OD	+0.75 –0.50 × 85 ($20/20^{+1}$)
	OS	+0.25 –0.25 × 80 (20/20)

Tentative Add at 40 cm: +1.00 diopters (20/20)

Phorometry (w/SRx):	**6 m**	**40 cm (w/+1.00 D add)**
Phoria	ortho	3^{Δ}XP'
BI vergence	X/9/4	24/26/22
BO vergence	X/16/10	24/32/16
Negative Relative Accommodation (NRA)/Positive Relative Accommodation (PRA)		+1.50/–1.25

Binocular Crossed-Cylinder Add at 40 cm: +1.25 D

Amplitude of Accommodation (w/o Rx): 3.50 diopters OD, 3.50 diopters OS, 4.00 diopters OU

Ocular Health, Tonometry and Visual Fields: Normal OU
Trial Frame: J.M. appreciated the slight improvement in distance vision with the subjective refraction data. She also responded favorably to her near vision with a +1.00 D add over the subjective refraction data.

Assessment
1. J.M.'s symptom of blurred vision at near was due to an uncorrected low hyperopia and astigmatism OU (OD > OS). That is, her habitual prescription contained only the +1.00 D add and not the additional plus needed to correct the hyperopia or the cylinder to correct the astigmatism.
2. Incipient presbyopia

Treatment Plan
1. Rx: OD   +1.75 –0.25 × 85
         OS   +1.50 –0.25 × 80

   Lenses were prescribed for near activities only, as the patient requested. When given the option of a multifocal lens or a second prescription for distance, the patient opted to continue with a prescription for near only.
2. Lens Design: Hard resin (CR-39) single vision lenses
3. Patient Education: J.M. was told that the new prescription would improve near vision and actually decrease distance vision because of the additional plus. The lenses would have to be removed for distance viewing. Re-examination in 12 to 18 months was recommended.

Discussion
The prescription for J.M. contained her subjective refraction data combined with a +1.00 D add in single vision form. The treatment options for a patient with ametropia (whether high or low) and presbyopia include: (1) a single near prescription only; (2) a single vision near prescription and a single vision distance prescription; and (3) a multifocal lens. J.M. chose the first option because she was used to a single vision prescription for near and only desired an update of this prescription. She felt that her distance vision did not warrant the inconvenience of an additional prescription for distance or a multifocal lens.

Often patients with low ametropia, when given the option of correcting the ametropia to improve visual acuity, elect to continue without the correction because they feel the slight improvement gained from a distance prescription is not enough to warrant wearing the lenses. For J.M., the chief complaint related only to near vision. However, the clinician has a responsibility to each patient to discuss and demonstrate the various options and to allow patients to make informed decisions that are best for them. The fact that uncorrected ametropia is present, especially if a low amount, does not in itself justify a correction.

Patient J.B.

History: J.B., a 15-year-old boy, presented stating that "Reading gets blurry after about 10 minutes." He reported that he had to blink and rest his eyes before he could continue reading. J.B. also noticed that after reading for a while, his distance vision seemed a little blurry. Squinting helped him see more clearly at distance. J.B. said he had no difficulty seeing the chalkboard in his classroom and that he had no headaches associated with reading. J.B.'s academic performance was at the B and C level. He liked sports, soccer and basketball in particular, and socializing with friends.

J.B. had never worn glasses or contact lenses. His last eye examination was 1 year before the current visit. His personal and family histories were otherwise unremarkable. He had been taking no medications.

Clinical Findings		6 m	40 cm
Habitual VA:	OD	20/20	20/20
	OS	20/20	20/20
Cover Test (w/o Rx):		1$^\Delta$XP	6$^\Delta$XP'
NPC: 3 cm			
Stereo Acuity at 40 (w/o Rx): 20 seconds (Randot)			
Keratometry:	OD	44.50/44.25 at 180° (with-the-rule)	
	OS	44.75/44.25 at 180° (with-the-rule)	
Retinoscopy:	OD	+0.50 DS	
	OS	+0.25 –0.25 × 180	
SRx:	OD	+0.50 DS (20/20)	
	OS	plano –0.50 × 180 (20/20^{+2})	

Phorometry (w/SRx):	6 m	40 cm
Phoria	2$^\Delta$XP	6$^\Delta$XP'
BI vergence	X/8/4	X/12/8
BO vergence	X/12/6	X/14/4
NRA/PRA		+2.50/–2.75

Amplitude of Accommodation: 6.00 diopters OD, 6.00 diopters OS, 6.50 diopters OU

Trial Frame: The subjective refraction data (SRx) were demonstrated with trial lenses in a trial frame at distance and near. J.B. noticed little difference in his vision at distance but did report that printed material at near appeared bolder and more distinct. After reading printed material for 10 to 15 minutes through the trial lenses, J.B. reported no blurring of the print and a feeling of greater comfort. He also noticed that after he read for this period of time, his distance vision through the prescription remained clear.

Retinoscopy with Cycloplegia (1% cyclopentolate): OD +0.75 DS, OS +0.25 −0.25 × 180

Assessment

1. J.B. manifested uncorrected simple hyperopia in the right eye and simple myopic astigmatism (with-the-rule) in the left eye. The amount of anisometropia in the vertical meridians was 1.00 diopter and that in the horizontal meridians was 0.50 diopter.
2. J.B. exhibited lower amplitudes of accommodation and a lower PRA add than expected for his age. These correlated findings suggested a possible dysfunction of accommodation. Vergences at far and near were low but indicated adequate compensation for the low phorias at the respective distances.
3. A cycloplegic objective refraction showed little difference from the noncycloplegic refraction, indicating the absence of latent hyperopia.

Treatment Plan

1. Rx: OD   +0.50 DS
   OS   plano −0.50 × 180
2. Lens Design: Polycarbonate single vision lenses
3. Patient Education: J.B. and his parents were informed of the nature of J.B.'s ametropia as the most likely cause of his symptoms when reading. He was instructed to wear the lenses as much as he felt was necessary but particularly for all nearpoint tasks. A reexamination in 1 year was recommended.

Discussion

J.B.'s symptom of blurred vision at near after a short period of reading was likely due to his inability to compensate for his uncorrected ametropias equally by accommodating, because a meridional anisometropia was present. Ultimately, accommodation fatigued and blur resulted. The only resolution of this inequality is corrective lenses. Because the prescription corrected for J.B.'s distance ametropia and provided normal visual acuity at far distances, the lenses could be worn full time as well as part time for reading only.

The lens-wearing habits of patients in cases of low ametropia are often at the patient's discretion, that is, when the person feels the need for corrective lenses. Young patients in particular, may become noncompliant if they are under the impression that they have to wear lenses full-time. On the other hand, if full-time wear is presented as optional, younger patients may be more likely to accept the correction, because they feel they have a choice. In J.B.'s case, full-time wear is truly optional.

Patient D.S.

History: D.S., a 43-year-old sales representative, presented with a symptom of some fatigue after a full day of near work. He had noticed that he became fatigued more quickly over the previous year. D.S.'s distance vision seemed quite good, although street signs at night were becoming difficult to read, especially after D.S. had worked a full day. D.S. had never worn spectacle or contact lenses. His general health was excellent and he had not been taking any medications. The personal and family histories were otherwise unremarkable.

Clinical Findings		6 m	40 cm
Habitual VA:	OD	20/20	20/30
	OS	$20/20^{-1}$	$20/20^{-2}$
Cover Test (w/o Rx):		ortho	$2^{\Delta}EP'$

Amplitude of Accommodation (w/o Rx): 5.00 diopters OD, 5.50 diopters OS
Stereo Acuity at 40 cm (w/o Rx): 20 seconds (Randot)

Keratometry:	OD	46.75/46.00 at 180° (with-the-rule)
	OS	46.25/45.25 at 10° (with-the-rule)
Retinoscopy:	OD	+0.75 DS
	OS	+0.50 DS
SRx:	OD	+1.00 DS (20/20)
	OS	+0.50 DS (20/20)

Phorometry (w/SRx):	6 m	40 cm
Phoria	ortho	$2^{\Delta}XP'$
BI vergence	X/10/6	12/18/8
BO vergence	12/20/10	
NRA/PRA		+2.50/–1.75

Binocular Crossed-Cylinder Add at 40 cm: +0.75 D
Ocular Health, Tonometry and Visual Fields: Normal OU
Trial Frame: The subjective refraction data were demonstrated in a trial frame so that D.S. could appreciate the slight improvement in visual acuity, especially at near, and the potentially improved comfort during reading. He was given the opportunity to read a magazine for 10 to 15 minutes to demonstrate comfort. He did notice a small improvement in acuity and comfort.

Assessment

1. Simple hyperopia OU (OD > OS) and anisometropia caused additional stress on the accommodation system, resulting in fatigue after prolonged nearpoint activities. The nighttime blur was also a result of accommodation fatigue, that is, the inability to compensate for the uncorrected hyperopia.
2. Low amplitudes of accommodation bordering on presbyopia. The amplitude OD was lower than OS because of the higher uncorrected simple hyperopia of the former.

Treatment Plan

1. Rx: OD +0.75 DS
        OS +0.25 DS
2. Lens Design: Hard resin (CR-39) single vision lenses
3. Patient Education: D.S. was advised of his uncorrected hyperopia and the reasons for his symptoms, especially at near point. It was further explained that because the symptoms were mild, there was not an urgency for corrective lenses. D.S. was given the option of holding off on the prescription and returning when he felt the necessity.

Discussion

Treatment of patients who have borderline vision problems is often successful because whether or not corrective lenses are prescribed, the patient is usually satisfied. The most important management tool in these cases is communication. Patients very much appreciate an explanation of their problem and reassurance that it is not serious and will not lead to something more serious.

When patients with low uncorrected ametropia and mild symptoms are presented with the option of corrective lenses or continuing as they have been, they often opt for the former and usually are satisfied with their decision. The responsibility of the clinician is to explain the options to the patient, including pro's and con's, and let the patient make the decision.

Patient T.C.

History: T.C., a 12-year-old girl, presented symptoms of a little blurred vision and frontal headaches when reading with her current spectacle lenses (HRx), which she had obtained 1 year earlier. She said that her glasses did not seem to be much better than no glasses at all. She did not notice the headaches on weekends or vacations from school.

T.C. was in 7th grade and a good student. She liked to read, but it was difficult for her. T.C. also liked sports such as soccer and softball.

She was in good health and taking no medications. The personal and family histories were otherwise unremarkable.

Clinical Findings		6 m	40 cm
Uncorrected VA:	OD	$20/25^{-2}$	$20/20^{-3}$
	OS	$20/25$	$20/20^{-1}$
Habitual VA:	OD	$20/25^{+1}$	$20/20^{-1}$ with +0.75 DS
	OS	$20/20^{-2}$	$20/20^{-1}$ with +0.50 DS
Cover Test (w/HRx):		2^{Δ}XP	8^{Δ}XP'

NPC: 15 cm

Stereo Acuity at 40 cm (w/HRx): 70 seconds (Randot)

Retinoscopy:	OD	$+0.50 - 0.50 \times 95$
	OS	$+0.50 - 0.50 \times 100$
SRx:	OD	$+0.50 - 0.75 \times 95$ ($20/20^{+2}$)
	OS	$+0.50 - 0.50 \times 100$ ($20/20^{+1}$)

Phorometry (w/SRx):	6 m	40 cm
Phoria	ortho	8^{Δ}XP'
BI vergence	X/8/5	8/18/14
BO vergence	8/16/10	6/10/4
NRA/PRA		+1.50/–1.00

Amplitude of Accommodation (w/SRx): 3.50 diopters OD, OS, OU

Trial Frame: The subjective refraction data were demonstrated in a trial frame. T.C. reported that her vision was clearer at distance and near. After reading for about 15 minutes with the trial lenses, T.C. felt a pulling sensation and pain at the front of her head.

Assessment

1. Low mixed astigmatism (against-the-rule) OD and simple hyperopic astigmatism (against-the-rule) OS. The uncorrected astigmatism OU is the likely cause of slightly blurred vision at far and near with the habitual prescription.
2. Convergence insufficiency as indicated by the moderate exophoria at near, low compensating (BO) vergence at near, low NRA add, and poor NPC. The condition likely contributed to the frontal headache T.C. experienced when reading.

Treatment Plan

1. Rx: OD $+0.50 - 0.75 \times 95$
   OS $+0.50 - 0.50 \times 100$
2. Lens Design: Polycarbonate untinted single vision lenses
3. Vision therapy for convergence insufficiency
4. Patient education: T.C. and her parents were informed of the prescription change and the condition of convergence insufficiency

as the likely causes of the symptoms T.C. experienced when reading. The need for a prescription change to maximize visual acuity and the need for vision therapy to enhance comfort and efficiency at near were emphasized. T.C. was instructed to wear the lenses for distance and near viewing (especially for reading). She was told that she could remove the lenses for physical activities if she so desired.

Discussion

This case illustrates the presence of more than one condition that contributes to a patient's symptoms. It is important that the clinician review the case history to attempt to identify an association between symptoms and vision activities. With T.C., the symptoms were not present when the particular task, that is, reading, was not performed. Therefore, the symptoms were very likely to be vision-related. It is possible that T.C.'s symptoms of blur and headache at near could have been attributed to the uncorrected astigmatism alone. However, other causes are possible, and they certainly should be explored. A convergence insufficiency is likely to cause such symptoms. Even though the stress on the vergence system is quite high for these patients, thus yielding a headache, the accommodation system also is compromised, yielding the symptom of blur.

The treatment plan for T.C. emphasized the maintenance of clear, comfortable, and efficient vision. The prescription and vision therapy each would address a different diagnosis, but both would contribute to the objective of the treatment plan.

Summary

The diagnosis and refractive management of low ametropia can be quite challenging to the clinician. Patients with low uncorrected ametropia often present with vague or transient symptoms, which can compromise a definitive diagnosis. Taking a thorough case history and conducting appropriate clinical tests are important to help identify other contributing factors, such as accommodation and vergence dysfunction, and to rule out other potential etiologies.

Typical symptoms resulting from these ametropias (low myopia, hyperopia or astigmatism) are blurred vision at distance or near, asthenopia, and asthenopic headache. These symptoms are certainly not unique to low ametropia but could be caused by a variety of conditions. Often the association of the symptoms with a specific vision task is a useful diagnostic feature.

Treatment planning for patients with low ametropia is quite simple once the diagnosis is made. These patients often report immediate relief of their symptoms with corrective lenses and therefore are highly motivated to comply. Adaptation to corrective lenses is fairly rapid because of the low lens powers involved. Special lens designs are usually not necessary for these patients except perhaps if there are unique vocational or avocational needs.

References

1. Blume AJ. Low-power lenses. In: Amos JF, ed. *Diagnosis and Management in Vision Care.* Boston: Butterworth-Heinemann, 1987:239–246.

2. Daum KM, Good G, Tijerina L. Symptoms in video display terminal operators and the presence of small refractive errors. *J Am Optom Assoc* 1988;59:691–697.

3. Collins MJ, Brown B, Bowman KJ, Carkeet A. Vision screening and symptoms among VDT users. *Clin Exp Optom* 1990;73:72–78.

4. Collins MJ, Brown B, Bowman KJ, Caird D. Task variables and visual discomfort associated with the use of VDT's. *Optom Vision Sci* 1991;68:27–33.

5. Yeow PT, Taylor SP. Effects of long-term visual display terminal usage on visual functions. *Optom Vision Sci* 1991;68:930–941.

6. Gur S, Ron S. Does work with visual display units impair visual activities after work? *Doc Ophthalmol* 1992;79:253–259.

7. Giles GH. *The Principles and Practice of Refraction and its Allied Subjects.* 2nd ed. London: Hammond, Hammond, 1965:229–237.

8. Hamilton EE. The quarter dioptry cylinder: some testimony for. *Ann Ophthamol Otolaryngol* 1894;4:328–335.

9. White JA. The practical value of low-grade cylinders in some cases of asthenopia. *Trans Am Ophthalmol Soc* 1894;12:153–168.

10. Cholerton MB. Low refractive errors. *Br J Physiol Opt* 1955;12:82–86.

11. Nathan J. Small errors of refraction. *Br J Physiol Opt* 1957;14:204–209.

Case Study Exercises

For each case study, determine the diagnosis and develop a treatment plan. The clinical questions provided with each case may assist you by highlighting important aspects of the case.

Patient J.R.

History: J.R., a 32-year-old man, presents with no vision problems with his habitual prescription, which he received 2 years earlier. He does want a new frame and lenses. He reports that he wears his glasses only for driving and movies. J.R. is in good health and is taking no medications. His personal and family histories are otherwise unremarkable except for a mention of hypertension in his family.

Clinical Findings		6 m	40 cm
Uncorrected VA:	OD	$20/25^{-2}$	20/20
	OS	20/25	20/20
Habitual VA:	OD	$20/20^{+3}$ with $-1.00 -0.25 \times 180$	
	OS	$20/15^{-2}$ with $-0.75 -0.25 \times 180$	
Cover Test (w/HRx):		ortho	$2^{\Delta}XP'$
Stereo Acuity at 40 cm (w/o HRx): 20 seconds (Randot)			
NPC: 2 cm			
Keratometry:	OD	43.50/42.75 at 170°	
	OS	44.00/43.00 at 175°	
Retinoscopy:	OD	-0.50 DS	
	OS	$-0.25 -0.25 \times 180$	
SRx:	OD	$-0.50 -0.25 \times 175 \ (20/20^{+3})$	
	OS	-0.50 DS $(20/15^{-1})$	

Phorometry (w/SRx):	6 m	40 cm
Phoria	ortho	ortho'
BI vergence	X/10/6	12/24/16
BO vergence	X/16/10	18/28/20
NRA/PRA		+2.25/–3.00

Clinical Questions
1. Do either the habitual prescription or the subjective refraction data correlate with the patient's uncorrected visual acuity? That is, would you predict the visual acuity obtained based on the patient's refraction data?
2. Is a change in J.R's prescription indicated even if he has no problem with his habitual prescription?
3. Is it necessary for J.R. to wear his prescription for near activities?
4. What would be the appropriate treatment plan for this patient?

Patient D.F.

History: D.F., a 25-year-old woman, presents reporting headaches after about an hour of computer work. She describes her headache as a dull pain radiating from the front to the sides of her head. D.F. says she has to take frequent breaks to alleviate the pain. She isn't sure but she thinks the computer monitor is a little blurry at times. These symptoms have been occurring for about 3 months. D.F.'s previous eye examination was 5 years earlier. She is in good health and is taking no medications. Her personal and family histories are otherwise unremarkable.

Clinical Findings		6 m	40 cm
Habitual VA:	OD	20/20	20/20
	OS	20/20	20/20
Cover Test:		ortho	3^ΔXP′

Stereo Acuity at 40 cm: 20 seconds (Randot)

NPC: 3 cm

Keratometry:	OD	44.00/44.00
	OS	44.00/43.75 at 180°
Retinoscopy:	OD	+0.50 DS
	OS	+0.50 DS
SRx:	OD	+0.50 –0.25 × 120 (20/20^{+2})
	OS	+0.50 –0.25 × 40 (20/20^{+2})

Phorometry (w/SRx):	6 m	40 cm
Phoria	ortho	4^ΔXP′
BI vergence	X/8/4	X/16/12
BO vergence	X/10/4	X/12/6
NRA/PRA		+2.50/–2.25

Amplitude of Accommodation (w/SRx): 8.50 diopters OD, OS

Clinical Questions

1. What is the most likely cause of D.F.'s symptoms?
2. Would you expect the patient to appreciate a difference in her visual acuity and vision comfort with and without the subjective refraction data in place?
3. Is there a potential vergence dysfunction? If so, what are the indicators?
4. What would be the most appropriate treatment plan for this patient?

Patient R.C.

History: R.C., a 45-year-old fashion designer, presents with a symptom of increasing difficulty maintaining clear vision at near. Her work involves detailed fashion drawings, which are becoming less distinct. She says she has no difficulty reading magazines, books, or newspapers. R.C.'s distance vision seems fine. She has never worn corrective lenses, and her previous examination was 2 years earlier. R.C. is in good health and is taking no medications. Her personal and family histories are otherwise unremarkable.

Clinical Findings:

		6 m	40 cm
Habitual VA:	OD	20/20	20/30
	OS	20/20	20/30
Cover Test (w/o Rx):		ortho	3^ΔXP'

Amplitude of Accommodation: 5.00 diopters OD, OS

Keratometry:	OD	43.25/43.00 at 180°
	OS	43.00/43.00
Retinoscopy:	OD	+1.00 −0.25 × 180
	OS	+0.75 DS
SRx:	OD	+0.75 −0.25 × 180 (20/20^{+2})
	OS	+0.75 −0.25 × 175 (20/20^{+3})

Tentative Add at 40 cm: plano (20/20)

Phorometry (w/SRx):	6 m	40 cm
Phoria	1^ΔXP	4^ΔXP'
BI vergence	X/8/4	X/20/12
BO vergence	X/16/10	X/22/10
NRA/PRA		+2.50/−1.50

Binocular Crossed-Cylinder Add at 40 cm: +0.75 D

Clinical Questions

1. Are the patient's nearpoint symptoms a result of her uncorrected hyperopia alone?
2. Would this patient be considered to have presbyopia? What are the diagnostic indicators for presbyopia?
3. Are corrective lenses indicated for this patient? If so, should they be recommended for full-time (distance and near) or part-time (near only) wear? If for part-time wear, should the low cylinder be included in the prescription?
4. Would single vision or multifocal lenses be most appropriate for this patient? Considering the patient's age, occupation, and symptom, what type of lens do you believe the patient would most prefer?

Patient A.Z.

History: A.Z., a 10-year-old boy, presents because he failed a vision screening at school. He says his vision is "pretty good," although he notices some difficulty reading his teacher's handwriting on the chalkboard. A.Z.'s teacher has seated him close to the front of the class, which seems to help. A.Z. also reports that he sometimes has difficulty seeing things far away that others can see without a problem. He adds that his eyes get tired sometimes when he reads for a long time. This is his first vision examination. A.Z. is a good student and he likes all kinds of sports. He is in excellent health and is taking no medications. His personal and family histories are otherwise unremarkable.

Clinical Findings		6 m	40 cm
Habitual VA:	OD	20/30^{-2}	20/20
	OS	20/30	20/20
Cover Test:		ortho	ortho'
Stereo Acuity at 40 cm:	30 seconds (Randot)		
NPC: 3 cm			
Keratometry:	OD	44.00/43.50 at 180°	
	OS	44.25/43.50 at 180°	
Retinoscopy:	OD	−0.25 −0.25 × 180	
	OS	−0.50 DS	
SRx:	OD	−0.50 −0.25 × 180 (20/20^{+2})	
	OS	−0.50 DS (20/20^{+3})	

Phorometry (w/SRx):	6 m	40 cm
Phoria	2$^{\Delta}$EP	6$^{\Delta}$EP'
BI vergence	X/12/6	X/16/8
BO vergence	X/24/12	X/24/10
NRA/PRA		+2.25/−4.25

Binocular Crossed-Cylinder Add at 40 cm: +1.00 D
Amplitude of Accommodation: >10.00 diopters OD, OS

Clinical Questions

1. Is the magnitude of the patient's ametropia consistent with his uncorrected visual acuity?
2. Are the patient's symptoms sufficient justification for recommending corrective lenses?
3. Is there a concern about accommodation and vergence problems from the wear of corrective lenses. If so, what advice should be given to the patient and parents? Should the lenses, if prescribed, be for full-time wear?
4. What would be an appropriate treatment plan for this patient? If corrective lenses are recommended, would it be advisable to include the low cylinder OD if the prescription is for part-time wear?

7   Presbyopia

Daniel Kurtz

A Case Study of Presbyopia

History: M.P., a 46-year-old book editor, presented with a complaint of trouble focusing on reading material for the past few months. Her eyes became uncomfortable within 20 minutes of reading. The problem was somewhat alleviated when she held reading material at arm's length, but she preferred not to have to do this. She noticed that she could see satisfactorily up close if she removed her current glasses. When she did so, however, she had to hold reading material at an uncomfortably close distance.

As an editor who reviewed submitted manuscripts, M.P. did a great deal of reading every weekday. She was of normal stature and her arms were of normal length. It seemed that she would be most comfortable reading at a distance of 40 centimeters. Her personal and family histories were otherwise unremarkable. M.P. was taking no medications. Her last physical examination had been 2 weeks earlier.

Clinical Findings		6 m	40 cm
Habitual Visual			
Acuity (VA):	OD	20/20	20/30 with −4.50 DS
	OS	20/20	20/30^{+1} with −4.50 DS
Cover Test (w/HRx):		2$^{\Delta}$XP	7$^{\Delta}$XP′
Amplitude of Accommodation (w/HRx):		5.00 diopters OD, OS	
Keratometry:	OD	41.87/42.25 at 85° (with-the-rule)	
	OS	42.87/43.12 at 75° (with-the-rule)	
Retinoscopy:	OD	−4.50 DS	
	OS	−4.50 DS	

Subjective Refrac-
tion (SRx):   OD   –4.50 DS (20/20)
                 OS   –4.50 DS (20/20)
Tentative Add at 40 cm: +0.75 diopters (20/20)

Phorometry (w/SRx):	**6 m**	**40 cm (w/+0.75 D add)**
Phoria	3$^\Delta$XP	10$^\Delta$XP'
Base-in (BI) vergence	X/12/8	X/24/14
Base-out (BO) vergence	X/14/6	X/12/6
Negative Relative Accom-		
modation (NRA)/Positive		
Relative Accommodation (PRA)		+1.50/–2.00

Binocular Crossed-Cylinder Add at 40 cm: +1.00 D
Range of Vision (w/+0.75 D add): 20 to 56 cm
Trial Frame: A +0.75 DS was held over each lens of M.P.'s habitual distance prescription to demonstrate reading vision through an add. She reported clarity of the print but felt a pulling sensation after reading a short time.

Assessment
1. Simple myopia OU (OD = OS) and no change from habitual lenses
2. Early presbyopia
3. Mild convergence insufficiency due to a moderate exophoria at near and a low compensating BO vergence

Treatment Plan
1. Rx: OD   –4.50 DS   +0.75 D add
       OS   –4.50 DS   +0.75 D add
2. Lens Design: Hard resin (CR-39) multifocal lenses with a flat top 28 mm segment
3. Patient Education: M.P. was advised of the various options available to satisfy her near visual requirements. She had worn glasses since she was 8 years of age and expressed no interest in contact lenses. When given the option of conventional or no-line bifocal lenses, she said that she "just wanted to keep it simple." The patient was also advised of the convergence insufficiency, which worsened with the add in place. Vision therapy was recommended to enhance her convergence skills. M.P. was told that the problem would likely increase as presbyopia advanced.

Discussion
Although an add of +0.50 D would give M.P. a balanced NRA/PRA (that is, equal plus and minus adds, respectively), it is unconventional to give so small an add to a patient with beginning presbyopia. More-

over, M.P.'s near vision and her range of clear vision through the +0.75 D add were ideal, and therefore this add was prescribed.

M.P. would be a straightforward, uncomplicated example of a patient with early presbyopia except for her potential convergence insufficiency. The slight increase in exophoria at near through the +0.75 D add combined with a low BO vergence produced a mild symptom of "pulling" when M.P. read. It was expected, however, that the symptom would disappear once the patient adapted to wearing an add lens. However, vision therapy to enhance convergence skills of a patient with presbyopia must also be considered. Base-in prism for near only is also an option but is less desirable than vision therapy, because it is usually a short-term solution. Patients often adapt to wearing the prism, and symptoms reappear. It is difficult to provide prism for near only in multifocal form. A single vision reading prescription with prism would have to be the alternative.

Although symptoms of convergence insufficiency are surprisingly infrequent among the presbyopic population, the clinician must not ignore this potential clinical problem, especially if a patient has early presbyopia.

Defining Presbyopia

Presbyopia literally means "old eyes." The *Dictionary of Visual Science* defines presbyopia as, "A reduction in accommodative ability occurring normally with age and necessitating a plus lens addition for satisfactory seeing at near."[1,2] To the clinician, presbyopia means that, because of normal aging, the amplitude of accommodation is no longer sufficient to meet the patient's functional needs at near distances.

Accommodation is the mechanism that has evolved in humans to produce plus dioptric power within the eye to compensate for the minus dioptric power that emanates from nearby objects. Real objects in the real world can only be the source of minus, or diverging, rays of light. Consequently, accommodation has evolved with only the ability to produce plus power, which converges the diverging rays coming from near objects so they can be brought to focus on the retina. Presbyopia is not a disease, a pathologic condition, or an anomaly. It is an expected and inevitable concomitant of the physiologic, healthy aging process of humans.[3]

The onset of presbyopia is not a function of the amplitude of accommodation or of the demand on the patient's accommodation. It is a function of the relation between the two.[4] "Insufficient" accommodation means that the person's ability is not great enough to satisfy his or her individual needs. Thus, a person with a larger than normal need to accommodate, such as someone with a 25-cm near working distance rather than the usual 40-cm distance, experiences presbyopia at an earlier age than the average person. A patient whose ability to accommodate declines at a slower rate than normal begins to experience presbyopia at a later age than the population norm.

Symptoms and Signs of Presbyopia

Patients with presbyopia typically present with complaints of blurry vision at near or with ocular discomfort and fatigue after fairly brief periods of near work.[2,5] At the onset of presbyopia, patients may report that they place reading materials on a low table and stand up to read until they are so far away that the letters are simply too small to recognize. Many patients literally complain that their "arms are too short." This occurs because, as ability to produce plus power within the eye declines, the person's first instinctive attempt to compensate involves holding the object of regard farther away, thus reducing the need to accommodate. By holding objects farther away, the person renders his or her reduced accommodative ability sufficient for the reduced demand, until even at arm's length the objects are too close. After realizing that they are unable to hold objects any farther away because of their physical limits, these patients seek professional help.

In presbyopia, symptoms are associated exclusively with near work. If the patient also has a problem with distance vision, there might be uncorrected ametropia in addition to presbyopia. For example, patients with hyperopia experience distance blur when their amplitude of accommodation is no longer adequate to compensate for the hyperopia. The diagnosis is then hyperopia, not presbyopia.

It follows from the foregoing discussion that the onset of presbyopia depends both on the *amplitude* of accommodation, which can be measured clinically, and on the patient's *demand* for accommodation, which must be assessed by a careful case history that covers when and how the patient views near stimuli. These two variables, amplitude and demand, also have a powerful influence on the management of the patient's presbyopia.

Common symptoms and signs associated with presbyopia are as follows:

1. Symptoms of blur at near or increased working distance for clearest vision at near
2. Decreasing visual acuity at near if ametropia at distance is fully corrected
3. Decreasing amplitude of accommodation, usually below 5.00 diopters.
4. Increasing lag of accommodation, requiring increased plus or decreased minus at near for normal visual acuity

5. Increasing exophoria or decreasing esophoria at near, although some patients with a large accommodative convergence/accommodation (AC/A) ratio manifest esophoria in early presbyopia
6. Decreasing positive relative accommodation add
7. Absence of a blur point during base-out and base-in vergence measurements at near

Prescription Considerations and Guidelines

At first the management of presbyopia seems trivial. Because an insufficiency of accommodation means that the patient is unable to generate enough plus power to meet near needs, one simply prescribes additional plus power over and above the distance prescription. The treatment of patients with presbyopia, however, involves a number of challenges, which center on two broad issues: (1) how much plus to prescribe, and (2) what form the plus should take.

The technical process of determining an add is described in detail elsewhere.[2-4] The focus of this chapter is the clinical thought process and the questions and issues the clinician must consider in deciding the add to prescribe. Many variables influence how much plus to prescribe. These variables cluster around two concepts—amplitude of accommodation and need (demand) for accommodation.

Amplitude of Accommodation

Measuring the amplitude of accommodation provides one starting point for determining the amount of additional plus needed at near. One standard clinical formula holds that patients can work comfortably for long periods of time if they sustain the use of no more than one-half of their total amplitude.[4]

Clinically, one can measure the amplitude by means of any of several accepted procedures.[2,3] If the patient can use at least 50 percent of the amplitude comfortably, the additional plus power required at near to satisfy the patient's needs (once these needs are identified) can be easily calculated in diopters. However, the assessment of these needs is not a trivial task.

On average, the single most important variable in predicting a patient's amplitude of accommodation is age.[2,6] Hofstetter performed an analysis and comparison of the amplitude versus age data of Donders and Duane[7] and derived formulas for determining the predicted minimum, maximum, and mean amplitudes as a function of age.[8] Table 7.1 shows the amplitudes of accommodation at various ages as determined with Hofstetter's formulas.

Other studies have shown that the amplitude declines gradually and inexorably with advancing age.[2,6,9,10] These studies agree that by the time the average patient reaches the sixth decade of life, he or she

TABLE 7.1   Predicted Amplitude of Accommodation as a Function of Age

| Age | Amplitude of Accommodation (Diopters)* | | |
	Minimum	Mean	Maximum
10	12.5	15.5	21.0
20	10.0	12.5	17.0
30	7.5	9.5	13.0
40	5.0	6.5	9.0
50	2.5	3.5	5.0
60	0.0	0.5	1.0
70	0.0	0.0	0.0

*Minimum amplitude = 15.0 D − (0.25 × age in years)
 Mean amplitude = 18.5 D − (0.30 × age in years)
 Maximum amplitude = 25.0 D − (0.40 × age in years)

can be expected to have an amplitude of accommodation of near zero diopters. Some studies have found the age at which most patients reach an amplitude of zero to be much younger.[11] The clinician cannot rely on studies but must treat each patient as an individual and determine the amplitude of accommodation at the time of the examination.

A variety of diseases of the eye, of the body, and of the mind may influence the patient's amplitude of accommodation and therefore the amount of plus needed for near vision.[2,12] Certain diseases can coexist with true presbyopia and influence the amount of plus power that the clinician needs to prescribe for near. For example, patients who have been treated with panretinal photocoagulation, usually to minimize the retinopathy associated with diabetes mellitus, may suffer damage to the long ciliary nerves. These nerves enter the eye near its equator, carry postganglionic parasympathetic fibers for accommodation, as well as for pupillary constriction, and may be inadvertently damaged when the retina is burned.

Any pathologic condition that results in permanent damage to the parasympathetic axons of the oculomotor nerve or the postganglionic fibers leads to a reduction in the amplitude of accommodation. In addition, diseases that affect the anterior uvea may involve the ciliary body, reducing its ability to produce accommodation. Moreover, a variety of medications have anticholinergic actions; that is, they may partially or totally block the neuromuscular junction at the ciliary body, reducing the amplitude of accommodation. If a patient has a lower than expected amplitude of accommodation for his or her age, all relevant diseases and medications must be considered.

Accommodation Demand: Assessing the Need

If a patient's distance prescription is inaccurate, the error will influence the patient's accommodation demand. For example, a patient with 3.00 diopters of hyperopia wearing a +2.00 diopter lens will have to accommodate not only near objects but also to overcome the 1.00 diopter of hyperopia that is not corrected. The following discussion presumes that any refractive error is fully corrected.

The total need for plus power at near depends on the distance between the patient's eye and the object of regard. Optometrists assume that the average patient views near objects from a distance of 40 cm. If the patient's vision is uncorrected, light rays from objects at 40 cm arrive at the eyes with a divergence of 2.5 diopters. To bring these rays to focus on the retina, the patient needs a total of 2.5 diopters of plus power, derived from the sum of accommodation and the plus add of the near prescription. However, if the patient is wearing a correction for distance or does not customarily work at a distance of 40 cm, the demand on accommodation will be other than 2.5 diopters.

The distance at which a patient usually works is sometimes called the *customary near working distance.* This distance has a powerful influence on the accommodation demand and is affected by the following factors.

1. *Patient Stature.* Conventional wisdom holds that persons of large stature and long arms will be comfortable viewing near objects from a distance greater than 40 cm, whereas people with short arms will be comfortable holding objects closer than 40 cm from their eyes. Thus, the length of the patient's arms, which generally correlates with the overall size of his or her skeleton, should influence the customary near working distance and thus the power of the add. However, some studies call this conventional wisdom into question.[13]

2. *Customary Near Tasks.* People use their eyes in different ways and engage in a variety of near tasks. Newspapers and books contain print that can be seen by most people from a distance of 40 cm. Telephone books and stock market reports, however, contain small print that many people want to hold at a distance closer than 40 cm. In contrast, most knitting tasks can be accomplished with a viewing distance of 50 cm. People who work all day with fine print typically hold the material closer than 40 cm and consequently have a much greater need for plus than people who work in front of a computer screen with a viewing distance of 60 cm.

Consequently, the clinician must carefully determine the tasks for which the patient will be using his or her near prescription and note anything out of the ordinary.[13] Because most people engage in a variety of near tasks, this assessment can be complex. Often the clinician must make a judgment about the average task and the average distance at which the patient works and prescribe accordingly.

Some patients may require different near prescriptions for different tasks.

3. *Vocational and Avocational Considerations.* "Some 30 percent of astronauts have described a loss in their ability to see objects clearly at close range when in space. Interestingly enough, most of the astronauts experiencing this change were in their early 40's and could see clearly without reading glasses when they were on the ground."[14]

Some jobs or hobbies may entail unusual visual or physiologic conditions that can affect the dioptric demand on the accommodation system, the patient's ability to accommodate, or both. The case of the astronauts who do not have presbyopia on earth but do have presbyopia in space illustrates this point, although the reason for their space-bound presbyopia is not known. Even for patients whose lives are more mundane than those of the astronauts, one should think about possible unusual conditions when making the final decision about how much plus to prescribe. Musicians who play in an orchestra, for example, generally view their music from a distance of about 50 to 80 cm but may read at the normal distance of 40 cm. These people need different add powers for working and reading.

4. *The Patient's Ametropia and Lens Effectivity.* When patients wear their correction in the form of contact lenses, their accommodation functions like that of a person with emmetropia. However, when vision is corrected with spectacles, the magnitude of the correction and its distance from the eye have powerful effects on the accommodation demand.

Patients with myopia experience presbyopia later than and need less plus than patients with hyperopia. Because of the way light rays pass through ophthalmic lenses, the actual physiologic stimulus to accommodation at the principle plane of the eye is fewer diopters for patients with corrected myopia than for those with corrected hyperopia even for the same viewing distance. Insofar as the amplitude of accommodation declines regardless of the patient's ametropia, patients with myopia need an add at a later age than patients with hyperopia, even if the ametropia of a person with hyperopia is fully corrected. For the same reason, patients with spectacle-corrected myopia need smaller adds, on the average, than age-matched patients with spectacle-corrected hyperopia.

One of the consequences of lens effectivity is that for a patient with spectacle-corrected myopia, the stimulus to accommodation declines with increases in the vertex distance of the distance correction (Table 7.2). One consequence of this phenomenon is that people with corrected myopia can aid their near vision through their distance eyeglasses by increasing the vertex distance. Without understanding the theory, some patients discover this for themselves, sliding their glasses farther and farther down their noses as their need for plus at near

TABLE 7.2 **Stimulus to Accommodation at the Eye as a Function of Spectacle Correction (Rx) and Vertex Distance (V) for a Target at 40 Centimeters**

Distance Rx (Diopters)*	Stimulus to Accommodation (Diopters)†		
	V = 14 mm	V = 27 mm	V = 40 mm
−15.00	1.72	0.00	0.00
−10.00	1.93	0.68	0.00
−7.50	2.05	1.20	0.50
−5.00	2.19	1.69	1.26
−3.00	2.31	2.05	1.81
−2.00	2.37	2.21	2.07
−1.00	2.43	2.36	2.30
plano	2.50	2.50	2.50
+1.00	2.57	2.62	2.67
+2.00	2.64	2.73	2.81
+3.00	2.72	2.81	2.91
+5.00	2.88	2.90	2.94
+7.50	3.11	2.84	2.56
+10.00	3.36	2.51	1.47
+15.00	3.97	0.53	0.00

*Refraction at a vertex distance of 14 mm.
†Calculated at the corneal plane.

gradually increases. This little trick allows them to function with their distance glasses for a little longer than their amplitude of accommodation should allow. However, just as at the onset of presbyopia patients feel that their arms are too short, now they may find that their nose has become "too short" to hold their glasses far enough away from their eyes for the glasses to continue to work well. When this occurs, it is time to prescribe an add or to increase the plus power at near.

Persons with low to moderate hyperopia (up to about 5 diopters) experience the opposite phenomenon. Increases in vertex distance produce a greater need for these patients to accommodate. However, people with higher hyperopia, like those with corrected myopia, also benefit from increases in vertex distance, as shown in Table 7.2. The calculations are based on the assumption that the stimulus to accommodation takes place at the corneal plane, an assumption that is approximately true for most eyes but does not hold for aphakic eyes.

The physiologic stimulus to accommodation is less through minus lenses than through plus lenses. This is true, however, only for lenses with a considerable vertex distance. Contact lenses can be thought of as having a vertex distance of zero. For this reason, a person with corrected myopia wearing spectacles has a lesser need to accommodate than the same patient wearing the correction in the form of contact lenses. Of course, the assumption is that the contact lens prescription is properly adjusted for the vertex distance. For example, compare the stimuli to accommodation through spectacles shown in Table 7.2 with 2.50 diopters, which is the comparable stimulus to accommodation through properly prescribed contact lenses. For the same reason, a person with myopia wearing contact lenses needs a higher add than a patient with myopia matched for age and ametropia wearing spectacle lenses. Similarly, contact lens wearers with myopia begin to experience presbyopia at an earlier age than patients with myopia that is corrected with eyeglasses. Moreover, many prepresbyopic individuals with myopia, when switching from spectacles to contacts, suddenly begin to experience symptoms of presbyopia. This is particularly true for persons with higher degrees of myopia.

The opposite holds true for patients with corrected hyperopia; that is, the contact lens wearer experiences presbyopia later and needs a smaller add than a patient of the same age with hyperopia and ametropia corrected with spectacles. Shifting the correction from the spectacle plane to the cornea, if the prescription is properly adjusted, eliminates the disadvantage of increased vertex distance.

Patients with anisometropia have different refractive errors in the two eyes.[1] If vision in both eyes is fully corrected, then the patient will be wearing different prescriptions over the two eyes. Because of lens effectivity, a difference in the demand on accommodation of the two eyes results when the patient looks at a near target. If the difference exceeds 0.12 diopter, the patient theoretically will require a different add power in each eye. Patients respond to anisometropia in a wide variety of ways,[15] and one should prescribe unequal adds only after testing them in a trial frame, not on the basis of theoretic considerations alone.

Visual Acuity and the Range of Clear Vision

In deciding how much plus to prescribe, the clinician must consider the patient's near visual acuity and the entire range of near distances over which the patient normally works. Visual acuity must be sufficiently good to meet the patient's need to recognize small visual stimuli at near. In the vast majority of cases, patients who can see 20/20 at 40 cm will be able to meet all their acuity needs.

In general, optometrists try to prescribe an add that will place the patient's customary near working distance at the dioptric midpoint of the range of clear vision, which is the range in space from the nearest point at which the patient can see clearly to the farthest point at which the patient can see clearly through the add. An add that requires a patient to use exactly half his or her amplitude of accommodation at the near working distance will achieve this goal. However, clinical measurements of the amplitude of accommodation are rarely precise enough to assure that this will occur. Consequently, one must always determine the customary near working distance and measure the linear range of clear vision from that reference point. If the far edge is not far enough away, then the add should be reduced. If the near edge of the range is too receded from the patient, then the add should be increased. Balancing these competing requirements constitutes one of the challenges of determining how much plus to prescribe.

When the add provides good vision and a good range of clear vision, then the patient will be able to function well with the add. Therefore, checking the visual acuity at near and the range of clear vision through the proposed add are the final, definitive tests to determine that the add is correct for the patient. All other means of determining the add are checked against the final outcomes of vision and range.[16]

Intermediate Blur

Many persons with advanced presbyopia experience what is called *intermediate blur.* For these patients there is a range of distances too far to be seen clearly through the add (beyond the range of clear vision) and too close to be seen clearly through the distance prescription because the amplitude of accommodation is too low. Intermediate blur results whenever the add exceeds the amplitude.

Prescribing a large add hastens the time at which a patient will likely experience intermediate blur.[15] For example, if one prescribes a +2.50 D add, then the far edge of the range of clear vision will extend beyond 40 cm by only the patient's depth of field. To see clearly beyond this distance, the patient will need to look through the distance correction and accommodate, which is precisely the kind of task for which the add was needed in the first place. For this reason, optometrists are generally "stingy" with the add, prescribing the lowest add that allows good function at near, and therefore delaying the time at which the patient experiences intermediate blur.

Eventually, however, the amplitude will decline to such a point and the add will have to be increased to such an amount that intermediate blur will be inevitable. If the intermediate blur is not acceptable, then the patient will need two different near prescriptions, one for close work and another for intermediate distances. Another option would be the use of progressive addition lenses (PALs).

Plus Adds and Exo Deviations

Whenever a patient looks through an add at near, accommodation will be less than that without the add for the same viewing distance. Because of the concurrent relaxation of accommodative convergence, the patient's near phoria will shift in a more exo or less eso direction. Optometrists take advantage of this phenomenon when they prescribe an add to relieve symptoms associated with overconvergence at near. In the case of patients with presbyopia, clinicians prescribe an add to substitute plus power in lenses for the plus that the patient can no longer generate from accommodation. However, the patient also gives up accommodative convergence when looking through the add. As a result, binocular posture through the add is less eso or more exo than the habitual posture. Patients with advanced presbyopia typically have large exophorias at near, and for most patients with presbyopia, the increase in exo deviation is usually not accompanied by any near symptoms.[17] However, some patients with presbyopia may experience fusional stress due to the increased exo posture. Because they cannot give up the add without also sacrificing near vision, these patients need both the add and vision therapy, or base-in prism, for their convergence insufficiency.[18]

Effects of Distance Prescription Changes on the Net Near Prescription

When the power of the distance prescription changes, the net near prescription (the power of the carrier plus the power of the add) may also change. If a patient's symptoms concern distance vision only (that is, near vision is satisfactory), then it is wise not to change the net near prescription. To maintain the net near prescription, the add power must be changed to compensate for changes in distance prescription power. For example, a patient presents with a –4.00 DS for distance and a +1.00 D add for near (that is, the net near power equals –3.00 DS). If the patient then needs a –4.50 DS to correct distance vision, an add of +1.50 D over the –4.50 DS carrier would be required to maintain the net near power of –3.00 DS.

In general, it is desirable to maintain the net near prescription for patients who are content with their habitual near correction. However, if preserving the net near power would require an add outside the usual add powers (that is, +0.75 D to +3.00 D), then one should allow the net near power to change in order to keep the add within the usual range. It is still advisable to keep changes in the net near power as small as possible, preferably +0.75 D or less.[4]

What is a "Normal" Add?

Adds less than +0.50 D, although useful for some purposes, rarely help patients with presbyopia. Adds greater than +3.00 D are special lenses usually reserved for patients with special needs due to reduced visual acuity, resulting from, for example, age-related maculopathy. Adds between +0.50 D and +3.00 D are very effective for the vast majority of patients with presbyopia.[16,19]

The Field of Vision

When selecting the form in which to prescribe the add, the clinician and the patient must not only consider working distance variables, which affect the amount of add required, but also must consider the parts of the visual field in which the patient will need to see up close and far away.[5] This is particularly true of spectacle wearers and is much less of an issue for contact lens wearers.

Objects viewed at distance through the near add will appear blurry. Thus, many wearers of conventional bifocals, which carry the add in the lower part of the lens, report difficulty descending stairs or stepping over curbs, since their feet are beyond their far point through the add and so are not seen clearly. Most patients adapt to these visual inconveniences, but some may not. All patients need to be educated about the possibility of perceptual problems when their vision is first corrected for presbyopia.

All bifocal lenses contain a transition between the distance and the near correction. The transition may be sudden, as in conventional spectacle bifocals, or it may be gradual, as in PALs. Nevertheless, all lenses contain such a transition, and as patients look into different parts of the visual field, they will move their direction of gaze through the transition point or points. When they do so, they will experience changes in image clarity, prismatic effects that produce image jump, or image distortions. Most but not all patients adapt to these perceptual irritations. All first time bifocal wearers must be warned of these effects before they start to wear their new correction.

Special bifocal designs are available for jobs and activities in which near viewing is directed toward parts of the visual field other than the usual position (converged and downward) or in which patients look down to see at distance. For example, custom-designed bifocals may be necessary for electricians, who look up to wire ceilings at arm's length, or golfers who look down to see the ball from a distance roughly equal to their height but who must also see the score card at the usual reading distance.

Problems with the visual field are associated with spectacle solutions to presbyopia. The contact lens options of monovision or simultaneous vision circumvent visual field problems.

Psychological Issues

Most patients do not share the professional's familiarity with age-related changes in the eyes and vision. When patients first become unable to see, even if the difficulty is limited to near viewing, they may become concerned that the problem is irremediable or will lead to blindness.[20] Full care should extend to addressing such anxieties with thorough patient education and reassurance therapy.[21]

Many patients fall victim to the "youth culture" of the western world. They correctly recognize that the need for reading glasses is concomitant with advancing age. In a vain attempt to avoid the inevitable, they deny to themselves and to others that they have a vision problem.[22] Alternatively, they may become upset at the realization. Kindness and gentleness can help patients overcome even these problems.

Some patients want to keep their visual problem invisible for a variety of reasons, such as not wishing to look middle-aged or simply not wanting to be seen in glasses even if just for reading. Such cosmetic concerns should be accepted as legitimate patient needs and be handled tactfully. Simple vanity is far from simple and has led many patients to choose contact lenses over eyeglasses.

Anisometropia

Anisometropia, because it can lead to different perceived image sizes between the two eyes, can affect the prescription options for presbyopia in several ways. Differences in image size present a barrier to fusion. In extreme cases, the patient may experience diplopia, and in less severe cases, asthenopia due to fusional stress. If the anisometropia is due to differences in corneal power, then contact lenses may reduce the fusional stress at distance, and a monovision fit for presbyopia may relieve fusional symptoms at near. On the other hand, if the anisometropia results from different axial lengths, then spectacle lenses will generally reduce fusional stress at distance. This option also will influence the means of correcting the presbyopia. These prescribing guidelines are based on Knapp's law.[5]

Patients with anisometropia that is fully corrected with spectacles experience induced vertical prism when they look down binocularly. Slab off prism may be used to compensate for unwanted vertical prism in bifocal spectacles. Having the patient use two pairs of glasses circumvents the problem. Use of contact lenses that do not involve translation of a lens on the cornea (simultaneous vision, monovision) also can be satisfactory.

Astigmatism

Some patients require a different correction for astigmatism when accommodating for near objects than when looking at distance because the eyes cyclorotate during near viewing.[2,15,23] Patients with high amounts of astigmatism are more at risk for this complication than other patients. For such patients, bifocal spectacles and most contact lenses will be troublesome; having two pairs of glasses with different cylindrical prescriptions, one for distance and one for near, may be the only satisfactory solution.

Spectacle Lens Treatment Options for Presbyopia

Multifocal Lenses

Benjamin Franklin receives credit as the inventor of bifocals for his realization that he could mount halves of lenses of two different powers in the same frame. He placed the lens for distance viewing in the top half of the eye wire and the lens for reading in the bottom half. The details of lens design have changed over the centuries, but the basic principle has not changed since Franklin's day. Stock bifocal lenses are available in a bewildering array of varieties, a catalog of which is beyond the scope of this chapter.

Bifocals cause some problems for patients. Because the near prescription stays on the patient's face, objects seen beyond the range of clear vision through the add appear unclear. Thus if the patient walks around with the bifocals on, curbs and stairs will usually be blurry. In addition, because of differences in prismatic effects between the carrier and the segment of the lens containing the add, there will be a sudden jump in target locations when the patient's gaze crosses the dividing line between the carrier and the add. These visual problems are intrinsic to bifocals; for some patients they are insurmountable barriers to acceptance of the lens design, and alternatives must be sought.

Patients who experience difficulty with intermediate blur may require trifocal lenses. The power for intermediate viewing is usually located just above the part of the lens that contains the reading add. In general, trifocal spectacles have the same benefits and disadvantages as bifocal spectacles. Use of PALs, like use of trifocals, helps solve the problem of intermediate blur for some patients.

No-Line Multifocal Lenses

The two most common forms of no-line multifocal lenses are the blended bifocal and the PAL. Blended bifocals have a blurred transition between the carrier and the segment. In almost all respects, they function as standard bifocals, except that the blurred transition is not visible to the average person. Therefore, blended bifocals function like conventional bifocals but cosmetically appear to be single vision lenses. They are useful for patients who wish to avoid the visible lines that tell the world they are old enough to need reading glasses.

Progressive addition lenses are a special class of no-line multifocals. PALs contain what is referred to as a *corridor* that connects the distance portion or carrier of the lens with the near portion. The power of the add increases gradually within the corridor. By looking through different parts of the lens, from carrier, through corridor, to the segment that contains the full add, the patient can find the proper lens power for all working distances, thus avoiding intermediate blur. Unfortunately, finding just the right spot on the lens takes practice and a combination of eye and head position that may not be comfortable for the patient. In addition, in the construction of such lenses, peripheral distortions are introduced in the lower portion of the lens to the left and right of the add. These distortions cause visual discomfort for many patients, particularly when the person moves about. Some patients complain of sea sickness while trying to adapt to PALs. As a result, these lenses are not suitable for all patients.

Multiple Pairs of Glasses

One way to avoid the problems associated with bifocals or trifocals is for the patient to use two pairs of spectacles, one for distance and another for near work. A third pair of glasses can be prescribed for intermediate distances. This option for correcting presbyopia is successful as long as the patient functions at the distance for which the glasses are prescribed.

Should the patient view an object at a distance other than the distance for which the glasses were prescribed, the object will appear blurry. Some patients complain of the inconvenience of having to possess and carry more than one pair of glasses, or of needing the pair that was left behind at home or work. Some patients complain of the inconvenience of having to switch glasses when looking from near to distance or distance to near.

Contact Lens Treatment Options for Presbyopia

Bifocal Contact Lenses (Alternating Vision)

Alternating-vision contact lenses contain a carrier, which is the patient's distance correction, and a separate portion that contains the add for near viewing. "Window" bifocal contact lenses and multifocal progressive addition (aspheric) contact lenses are miniature versions of bifocal or PAL spectacles. The portion of the lens that contains the add occupies a small portion, or window, of the total lens. Unfortunately, lens rotation, a common feature of contact lenses, takes the add out of its proper position with respect to the line of sight. Concentric bifocal contact lenses, in which the add resides in an annulus around the entire periphery of the lens, circumvent the problem of rotation.[24]

For all types of alternating-vision contact lenses, the lens must sit on the cornea in the correct position to bring the add before the patient's line of sight during near tasks. Moreover, the translation must be of nearly equal amounts in both eyes. Translation is usually achieved by having the lower lid push the lens up when the patient looks down; however, the action of lid on lens is uncomfortable for some patients.[24]

Overcorrection of Contact Lenses with Reading Glasses for Near

Another solution to the problem of presbyopia that includes contact lenses is to fit the patient with lenses for distance and to fit the add in near-vision-only spectacles. In some ways this represents the worst and the best of both worlds. Visual function is good at all distances with this combination. On the other hand, the patient reveals his or her age, has the cosmetic problems associated with glasses, and suffers the inconveniences of wearing and having to carry spectacles. In addition, the patient experiences the risks associated with contact lens wear and the inconveniences of taking care of the lenses.

Simultaneous Vision Bifocal Contact Lenses

The patient fit for "simultaneous vision" views through the distance and the near prescriptions at the same time. One example of this type of contact lens is a concentric design in which the add occupies the center of the lens and is surrounded by the distance prescription. The patient simultaneously sees both a clear and a blurry image when looking either at distance or at near.[24] Under these conditions, the patient must learn to suppress the blurry image and attend only to the clear one. Such patients experience ghost images and reductions in visual acuity and contrast sensitivity. Because this type of contact lens also reduces illumination by about 20 percent, problems are exacerbated under dim conditions such as night driving.[25]

Monovision

Although theoretically applicable to spectacles as well as to contact lenses, monovision is an approach reserved almost exclusively for the latter.[26] In this option, one eye, usually the sighting dominant eye, is fit with its prescription for distance viewing and, at the same time, the fellow eye is fit with its prescription for near viewing (that is, the sum of the distance correction and the add). Monovision results in a slight drop in binocular visual acuity and contrast sensitivity both at distance and at near when compared with overcorrection with spectacle lenses for near only.[27]

Because for any given viewing distance, a patient fit with monovision must have blurry vision through one eye or the other, monovision presents a barrier to fusion. Therefore, a patient with monovision lenses with a fusional system on the verge of decompensation may experience diplopia or increased fusional stress and asthenopia. If, however, the patient is able to suppress the blurry image in either eye or lacks fusion, he or she should experience no such fusional stress and is a better candidate for monovision. Even with the best result, however, on theoretical grounds, monovision should cause a reduction in the patient's stereopsis, because clear vision in both eyes simultaneously can no longer be achieved. Functional problems with monovision, as with simultaneous viewing, are exacerbated in dim light, that is, scotopic viewing conditions.[28]

Both monovision and simultaneous-viewing contact lenses force the brain to deal with two images, either from the same eye or from the two eyes; one of these images is out of focus. In general, patients cope with this challenge by suppressing or ignoring the blurry image. Thus, any variable that makes such suppression more difficult will interfere with the patient's ability to succeed with these options. Eliminating peripheral cues and increasing the size of the add are examples of such variables.[27]

Contact lenses for distance combined with spectacle lenses for near seem to provide the best function among the various contact lens options for patients with presbyopia. This condition serves as the control condition in many of the studies evaluating various contact lens options for patients with presbyopia.[29] Monovision or simultaneous-viewing contact lenses provide more of the cosmetic advantages of contacts over spectacles and provide better function than other contact lens options for prebyopia.[27,30] However, they impair visual function to some degree in most patients.[31] The problems are worse under impoverished visual conditions and with higher add powers.[25] Alternating-vision (for example, window) contact lenses provide good appearance but may be less comfortable than single vision contacts and are susceptible to problems associated with lens movement, particularly rotation. The prudent clinician should thoroughly assess the patient's visual needs and functional status when a patient with presbyopia wants to wear contact lenses and help the patient to choose an option that addresses as many of the patient's needs as possible.

Case Studies of Presbyopia

Patient A.M.

History: A.M., a 48-year-old physician, presented with trouble focusing on reading material that had lasted for the past few months. The problem was somewhat alleviated when she held reading material farther away, but this was awkward and A.M. preferred not to have to do this. She had not undergone an eye examination since she was in medical school 18 years earlier and stated that she had always had perfect vision at all distances until the present. She was very emphatic about not wanting to appear middle-aged and "would not be bothered" with glasses. Nevertheless, as a physician, A.M. did a lot of reading every day. A.M. was of normal stature and her arms were of normal length, well suited for comfortable reading at a distance of 40 cm. Her personal and family histories were otherwise unremarkable. A.M. was in good health and taking no medications.

Clinical Findings		6 m	40 cm
Habitual VA:	OD	20/20	20/30^{-1}
	OS	20/20	20/30^{+1}

Amplitude of Accommodation (w/o Rx): 4.00 diopters OD, OS

Keratometry:	OD	44.75/44.50 at 85° (against-the-rule)
	OS	43.75/43.50 at 85° (against-the-rule)
Retinoscopy:	OD	+0.50 DS
	OS	+0.25 DS
SRx:	OD	plano sphere (20/20)
	OS	plano sphere (20/20)

Tentative Add at 40 cm: +1.00 D (20/20)

Phorometry (w/SRx):	6 m	40 cm (w/+1.00 D add)
Phoria	1$^\Delta$XP	2$^\Delta$XP'
BI vergence	X/12/10	12/16/10
BO vergence	16/14/8	18/22/14
NRA/PRA		+1.25/–1.75

Binocular Crossed-Cylinder Add at 40 cm: +1.00 D
Range of Vision (w/+1.00 D add): 20 to 70 cm
Ocular Health, Tonometry, and Visual Fields: Normal OU
Trial Frame: A +1.00 DS OU was demonstrated for reading only. A.M. was very impressed with the clarity of reading material and the range of vision. She was also made aware of the blurred vision at distance with the lenses.

Assessment
1. Emmetropia OU
2. Early presbyopia

Treatment Plan
1. Rx: OD plano sphere   +1.00 D add
       OS plano sphere   +1.00 D add
2. Lens Design: Options for this prescription were discussed, that is, single vision for near either full field or half eye, multifocal lenses (PAL in particular), and contact lenses (monovision or bifocal). Because of her concern for cosmesis and potential interference from a spectacle frame, A.M. opted for monovision contact lenses.
3. Patient Education: A.M. was instructed about the care and handling of the contact lenses during fitting and dispensing visits. She was encouraged to obtain single vision spectacle lenses for near as back-up.

Discussion
Finding the right amount of plus for A.M. was fairly easy. A minimal add of +1.00 D provided her with good acuity at near and a good range of clear vision. This add, however, did not balance the NRA and PRA (+1.25 D add would have balanced these findings), although

it was consistent with the binocular crossed-cylinder add. However, the lowest add that provides acceptable acuity and a good range of vision is the most desirable, especially for a first-time add wearer. An add higher than +1.00 D would be overkill in this case. The patient must also understand that the add will have to be increased periodically, although the frequency of change is uncertain.

A.M. had a slight amount of hyperopia. However, the correction of the hyperopia was rejected during the subjective refraction. For all practical purposes, A.M. was treated as having emmetropia. The issue with A.M. concerned the form of the plus add. When she arrived for her examination, she was emphatic about not wanting to wear glasses, so that option was considered as the last choice. On the other hand, A.M. had never worn contact lenses and was unaccustomed to their handling and care. Nevertheless, she was strongly motivated to try contact lenses. After appropriate patient education, monovision contact lenses were her choice. Bifocal contact lenses were an alternative that was considered but rejected by the patient. Although the contact lenses will likely be worn most of the time, patients need to be encouraged to obtain spectacle lenses in case the contact lenses are unwearable for any reason.

Patient P.P.

History: P.P., a 46-year-old engineer, presented with eyestrain after 30 minutes of near work and intermittent blur during near work in the evening. Almost all of his work involved close, detailed work. His hobbies were reading and working on Z-gauge model electric trains (the smallest kind). He often took off his glasses to work on the trains, holding them 15 to 20 cm from his eyes.

P.P. stated that he had always been concerned with his vision. He said that as a child he demanded that his glasses be updated often in order to preserve maximum acuity. He thought he had begun wearing glasses when he was 3 or 4 years of age and never had gone anywhere without them. P.P. once tried contact lenses but gave them up after 3 months because they gave him "eyestrain" and besides, he preferred wearing glasses. P.P.'s personal and family histories were otherwise unremarkable. P.P. was in good health and taking no medications.

Clinical Findings		6 m	40 cm
Habitual VA:	OD	20/20	20/20 with −2.25 −0.25 × 15
	OS	20/20	20/20 with −6.50 − 1.25 × 173
Stereo Acuity at 40 cm (w/HRx): 40 seconds (Randot)			
Amplitude of Accommodation (w/HRx): 5.00 diopters OD, OS			
Keratometry:	OD	41.25/41.87 at 80° (with-the-rule)	
	OS	44.75/46.50 at 85° (with-the-rule)	

Retinoscopy: OD   –2.50 DS
                    OS   –6.50 –1.25 × 175
SRx: OD   –2.50 DS (20/20^{+2})
                    OS   –6.50 –1.25 × 175 (20/20)
Tentative Add at 40 cm: +0.75 D (20/20)

Phorometry (w/SRx):	**6 m**	**40 cm (w/+0.75 D add)**
Phoria	2$^\Delta$EP	2$^\Delta$EP′
BI vergence	X/18/12	12/16/10
BO vergence	22/26/18	24/28/24
NRA/PRA		+2.00/–1.75

Binocular Crossed-Cylinder Add at 40 cm: +0.75 D
Ocular Health, Tonometry, and Visual Fields: Normal OU

Assessment

1. Simple myopia OD and compound myopic astigmatism (with-the-rule) OS
2. Anisometropia (4.0 diopters in the 180° meridian and 5.25 diopters in the 90° meridian)
3. Incipient presbyopia

Treatment Plan

1. Rx: OD –2.25 –0.25 × 15   +0.75 D add
        OS –6.50 –1.25 × 173   +0.75 D add with 3$^\Delta$ base-up prism
2. Lens Design: Hard resin (CR-39) multifocal lenses with a flat top 35 mm segment and 3$^\Delta$ of slab-off prism OS
3. Patient Education: P.P.'s ametropia and the need for a reading add and slab-off prism was explained to him. P.P. understood the cosmesis of the lenses and that adjustments to the new prescription would be required. The influence of direction of gaze through the spectacle lenses on comfort and efficient use also was explained.

Discussion

P.P. had refractive anisometropia; that is, the difference in ametropia between his eyes was due to differences in refractive power, probably not in axial length. This conclusion was supported by the keratometry readings and by the patient's report that a brief attempt to wear contact lenses resulted in eyestrain.

P.P. had 5.25 diopters of anisometropia in the vertical meridian. Therefore, when he looked 10 mm down for reading with his habitual spectacle lenses, 5.25 prism diopters of vertical imbalance in the direction of base-down prism over the left eye was induced. To offset this imbalance, base-up prism slabbed off over the left was prescribed. However, deciding exactly how much prism to prescribe is a challenge. In general, one must try to keep the amount of prism to the minimum necessary. P.P. would probably look down by different amounts for different occasions, thus inducing different amounts of prism each time. Moreover, as a patient with long-time anisometropia who showed no vertical imbalance, P.P. had learned to look through the optical centers of his lenses at all working distances by adjusting his head position. In his new bifocal lenses, P.P. would have to learn to look down, but not necessarily by 10 mm. By setting the top of the segment at his lower lid, P.P. should have been able to function with a modest amount of down gaze, about 6 mm. Therefore, the amount of prism needed in the prescription would likely be less than 5.25 prism diopters.

A method to determine the amount of prism in these cases would be to have the patient put on the habitual spectacle lenses, and then with the new add held over the lenses where the segment would be, introduce different amounts of prism until the patient reports comfortable vision. Even when this technique is used, there are some risks, because it is quite difficult to replicate the bifocal segments in this manner, and the circumstances in and duration with which the patient will use them.

Patient H.W.

History: H.W., a 54-year-old caterer, presented with trouble reading the unit pricing tags on the higher shelves at the supermarket for the previous few months. She could not seem to get far enough away to see them through the top of her glasses, though this is what she had been doing up to a few months previously. H.W. could read "adequately" through her bifocals but could not crane her neck far enough to use them for the upper shelves. As a caterer, she spent a great deal of time in the market. When questioned, H.W. also admitted that the stove top was looking a little blurrier than it used to.

Clinical Findings		6 m	40 cm
Habitual VA:	OD	20/25	20/40^{+2} with +1.00 DS
	OS	20/25	20/30^{-2} with +0.75 DS
			+2.00 D add OU
Keratometry:	OD	41.75/42.12 at 95° (with-the-rule)	
	OS	42.50/42.62 at 80° (with-the-rule)	
Retinoscopy:	OD	+1.25 DS	
	OS	+1.25 DS	
SRx:	OD	+1.25 DS (20/20)	
	OS	+1.25 DS (20/20)	
Tentative Add to 40 cm:	+2.00 D (20/20)		

Phorometry (w/SRx):	6 m	40 cm (w/+2.00 D add)
Phoria	ortho	9^ΔXP'
BI vergence	x/10/8	11/16/14
BO vergence	12/15/12	16/22/18
NRA/PRA		+0.50/–0.50

Range of Vision (w/+2.00 D add): 30 to 50 cm
Ocular Health, Tonometry, and Visual Fields: Normal OU

Assessment
1. Simple hyperopia OU
2. Presbyopia with intermediate blur

Treatment Plan
1. Rx 1: OD +1.25 DS   +2.00 D add
          OS +1.25 DS   +2.00 D add
   Rx 2: OD +2.00 DS   +1.25 D add
          OS +2.00 DS   +1.25 D add
2. Lens Design: Hard resin (CR-39) multifocal lenses with flat top 28 mm segments
3. Patient Education: Prescription 1 was for driving, reading, and bookkeeping. Prescription 2 was for shopping and cooking. H.W. was advised that the change in her prescription was normal and expected for her age. She was instructed on the use of the two bifocal prescriptions.

Discussion
H.W. had a classic case of presbyopia with intermediate blur. The conventional solution for such a patient is trifocals. However, H.W.'s vocational needs often placed objects at intermediate distances above the straight ahead position of gaze. The conventional placement of trifocals (that is, the top of the intermediate segment is placed at the lower margin of the pupil) would be of little help when she looked at the uppermost shelves. H.W. spent a substantial portion of her day in activities that demanded the intermediate range of vision. Therefore, it was worth her while to invest in a pair of vocational lenses, that is, a correction that was suitable only when she was shopping or cooking. This was achieved with bifocal lenses containing an intermediate-distance prescription in the carrier lenses and a full plus, near distance prescription in the segments. A second pair of lenses with the full distance correction on top and the full add in the segment would allow H.W. to perform all her other daily activities, such as driving, balancing the books for her catering business, and watching television.

A +2.00 D add provided a good range of clear vision and balanced the patient's NRA and PRA. This add was therefore prescribed for prescription 1. The +2.00 D carrier lens in prescription 2 represented an add of +0.75 D over the distance prescription. Through this add, the patient's far point was approximately 1.33 meters, which was a good working distance for shopping (for example, reading grocery prices). The total add of +2.00 D through the bifocal segment maintained the patient's ability to function at a 40-cm working distance. The 35 mm segments were chosen to provide a larger field of view than a more conventional 25 or 28 mm segment.

Patient L.L.

History: L.L., a 74-year-old woman, presented with trouble focusing on her needlepoint for a few months prior. She had also noticed that her distance vision was not as good as it used to be, but because she did not drive, it had not been a problem for her. L.L. had undergone a complete physical examination on her birthday 3 months earlier and was given a clean bill of health. L.L. had some trouble sleeping but had devised a successful self medication regimen of a tall glass of sherry mixed with warm milk just before going to bed. L.L.'s personal and family histories were otherwise unremarkable. She was taking no medications.

Clinical Findings		6 m	40 cm
Habitual VA:	OD	20/30^{-2}	20/40 with +2.25 −0.75 × 90
	OS	20/40	20/40 with +2.75 −1.25 × 100
			+2.50 D add OU
Keratometry:	OD	40.75/41.25 at 175° (against-the-rule)	
	OS	41.25/41.50 at 165° (against-the-rule)	
Retinoscopy:	OD	+3.00 −1.25 × 90	
	OS	+3.25 −1.25 × 90	
SRx:	OD	+3.00 −1.25 × 95 (20/30)	
	OS	+3.25 −1.00 × 100 (20/30)	

Tentative Add at 40 cm: +2.50 (20/30)

Phorometry (w/SRx):	6 m	40 cm (w/+2.50 D add)
Phoria	2$^\Delta$XP	14$^\Delta$XP′
BI vergence	X/11/8	8/11/5
BO vergence	8/13/10	11/17/9
NRA/PRA		+0.75/−0.25

Range of Vision (w/+3.00 D add): 25 to 35 cm
Ocular Health: 1$^+$ nuclear sclerotic cataracts in OD and OS. L.L. had dry eyes but had been successfully using tear replacement eye drops for 6 years. Internal examination was unremarkable OU.

Assessment
1. Compound hyperopic astigmatism (against-the-rule) OD and OS
2. Absolute presbyopia
3. Nuclear sclerotic cataracts OD and OS causing reduced visual acuity

Treatment Plan
1. Rx: OD +3.00 –1.25 × 95   +3.00 D add
   OS +3.25 –1.00 × 100   +3.00 D add
2. Lens Design: Hard resin (CR-39) multifocal lenses with flat top 35 mm segments
3. Patient Education: L.L. was advised about the need to hold reading material close (that is, at 30 cm with the new bifocal lenses), to use good lighting when reading, and about early cataracts. She was told that cataract surgery was not yet indicated because of her relatively good vision but that periodic monitoring of the cataracts was important. L.L. was advised to return in 1 year for a reexamination.

Discussion
Although L.L. reported no problems with her distance vision, a slight change in the distance prescription gave her slightly better vision. Moreover, the extra plus at distance also gave her more plus in the net near prescription. Increasing the add to +3.00 D gave L.L. even more plus at near. Although this forced L.L. to work at 30 cm rather than a more customary 40 cm, she had a small stature and preferred close distances when doing her needlepoint. The +3.00 D add improved L.L.'s near acuity and provided a reasonable range of clear vision. A flat top 35 mm segment was chosen because it provided a large area through which to work at near and made near vision less dependent on eye position as compared with a smaller segment.

Like the majority of patients her age, L.L. had cataracts that slightly impaired her vision. However, with the increased plus at near, L.L. could continue to enjoy her hobby and to function quite well. Cataract surgery was not yet needed because L.L. was able to function adequately with the visual acuity achieved from the new bifocal lenses.

Patient R.F.

History: R.F., a 42-year-old college professor, presented with trouble focusing on reading material for the few months prior. The patient's record showed that he had moderate myopia and had been fitted with contact lenses 9 years earlier. He insisted that the contact lenses were comfortable and that he saw "beautifully" at distance. R.F.'s habitual spectacle lens prescription (HRx 1) and contact lens prescription (HRx 2) were OD –4.25 DS and OS –4.50 DS.

R.F. was of normal stature. Because his job entailed a great deal of reading, R.F.'s hobbies involved no near work. He enjoyed swimming, playing tennis, and rock climbing. His personal and family histories were otherwise unremarkable. R.F. was in good health and was taking no medications.

Clinical Findings		**6 m**	**40 cm**
Habitual VA:	OD	20/20	$20/20^{-2}$ with –4.25 DS
	OS	20/20	$20/20^{-2}$ with –4.50 DS
Over-refraction			
(w/HRx 2):	OD	+0.50 DS (20/20)	
	OS	+0.50 DS (20/20)	

Amplitude of Accommodation (w/HRx 2): 4.00 diopters OD, OS

Keratometry		
(w/o HRx 2):	OD	45.25/44.50 at 70° (against-the-rule)
	OS	46.37/45.87 at 85° (against-the-rule)
Retinoscopy:	OD	–4.25 DS
	OS	–4.50 DS
SRx:	OD	–4.50 DS (20/20)
	OS	–4.75 DS (20/20)

Tentative Add at 40 cm: +1.25 D (20/20)

Phorometry (w/SRx)	**6 m**	**40 cm (w/+1.25 D add)**
Phoria	ortho	ortho'
BI vergence	11/12/8	14/16/12
BO vergence	14/22/18	22/26/14
NRA/PRA		+1.75/–1.50

Binocular Crossed-Cylinder Add at 40 cm: +1.25 D
Range of Vision (w/+1.25 D add): 25 to 70 cm
Ocular Health, Tonometry, and Visual Fields: Normal OU

Assessment
1. Simple myopia OU
2. Early presbyopia

Treatment Plan
1. Rx: No change in current contact lens prescription. Dispense a new pair of lenses. Prescribe single vision lenses for reading to use in conjunction with the contact lenses: OD +1.25 DS and OS +1.25 DS.
2. Lens Design: Hard resin (CR-39) single vision lenses

3. Patient Education: R.F. was advised about the need for an additional prescription for reading. The options, including monovision and bifocal contact lenses, were discussed and rejected by the patient.

Discussion
R.F. had begun to experience presbyopia at an earlier age than most patients because he was a contact lens wearer and because his contact lens prescription was slightly overminused. Because the patient was happy with his comfort and vision with the contact lenses, this prescription was left unchanged, at least for distance vision. An add of +1.25 D provided good acuity at 40 cm, a balanced NRA/PRA, and a satisfactory range of vision. This add was slightly higher than expected for a patient of R.F.'s age because the contact lens prescription was slightly overminused (over-refraction of +0.50 DS).

As far as his symptoms were concerned, it was important to advise R.F. of the various options available to solve his problem. R.F. was adamant that he wanted to retain his sharp distance vision with the contact lenses. He wanted to continue to look and feel young on the tennis courts. After considering monovision and bifocal contacts, R.F. decided that reading glasses over his contacts would work well for him. He could leave them on his desk at work, where he did all his reading. If his students caught him with them on, it would only make him "look more distinguished, not older," he said.

Patient M.G.

History: M.G., a 59-year-old insurance agent, presented with trouble focusing on reading material for the previous few months with the bifocal lenses prescribed 3 years earlier by the same clinician. He reported that he could read as long as he wanted without experiencing eyestrain. M.G. had also begun to notice that his distance vision, which used to be "perfect" was not quite as sharp as he would have liked. The patient's record indicated that he has low hyperopia, for which conventional flat top 28 mm bifocal lenses in plano carriers had been prescribed.

Clinical Findings		**6 m**	**40 cm**
Habitual VA:	OD	$20/25^{-1}$	20/40 with plano sphere
	OS	$20/25^{-2}$	$20/30^{-2}$ with plano sphere +1.75 D add OU
Keratometry:	OD	44.25/44.50 at 90° (with-the-rule)	
	OS	45.37/45.87 at 85° (with-the-rule)	
Retinoscopy:	OD	+0.75 DS	
	OS	+1.00 DS	

SRx: OD   +0.75 DS (20/20^{+2})
              OS   +0.75 DS (20/20^{+3})
Tentative Add at 40 cm: +1.50 D (20/20)

Phorometry:	6 m	40 cm (w/+1.50 D add)
Phoria	ortho	10$^{\Delta}$XP′
BI vergence	9/11/6	18/22/16
BO vergence	11/18/5	12/16/12
NRA/PRA		+1.00/–0.75

Range of Vision (w/+1.50 D add): 30 to 60 cm
Ocular Health: Unremarkable except for trace nuclear sclerosis of the crystalline lenses
Trial Frame: The subjective refraction data with a +1.50 D add were demonstrated to M.G. in a trial frame. He noticed a distinct improvement in his distance vision with the correction of +0.75 DS OU, and the add provided an acceptable range of clear and comfortable vision.

Assessment
1. Simple hyperopia OU (OD = OS)
2. Moderate presbyopia

Treatment Plan
1. Rx: OD   +0.75 DS   +1.50 D add
        OS   +0.75 DS   +1.50 D add
2. Lens Design: Hard resin (CR-39) bifocal lenses with a FT-28 mm segment
3. Patient Education: M.G. was advised of the change in his prescription and the need for a distance as well as near correction. He was also advised that a slight decrease in his range of vision through the add may occur because the total plus at near was increased by 0.50 diopter.

Discussion
M.G. had gone many years without wearing a refractive correction for his hyperopia. Between his depth of field and his accommodation, M.G. always had been able to compensate for the hyperopia. However, he then began to experience near-absolute presbyopia, and thus his small amount of hyperopia could not be compensated with the even smaller amount of accommodation. M.G. then started to notice that his distance vision was worsening.

   Prescription of a +1.50 D add, though smaller than the patient's habitual prescription, provided a total near power of +2.25 D, which was 0.50 diopter greater than his habitual. At first glance, the additional 0.50 diopter of plus may seem too small to improve acuity at near by three or so lines of letters. However, M.G. did achieve this improvement, as demonstrated with trial framing.

The changes in M.G.'s prescription were consistent with his entering symptoms and visual acuities. Because the changes were relatively small, M.G. would not be expected to experience any difficulty with adaptation. Using the same bifocal segment type helps facilitate adaptation for most patients.

Although M.G. demonstrated high exophoria at near through the new distance and near prescription, he did not experience any symptoms attributable to this phoria or convergence insufficiency. Thus no action was considered necessary to address the near phorometry findings.

Summary

When prescribing for presbyopia, clinicians must address two broad questions, that is, how much plus to prescribe for near, and in what form will the plus be prescribed?

In deciding how much plus to prescribe, the clinician must consider the patient's amplitude of accommodation. But the clinician must also consider variables that affect how much demand is placed on accommodation during the patient's daily life. The demand is determined by the patient's stature, customary near tasks, vocational and avocational needs, and ametropia. In assessing the patient's functional capability through the add, the clinician should assess the patient's visual acuity and the range of clear vision and should also consider the possibilities of intermediate blur, problems associated with an exo deviation, and the influence of changes in the distance prescription on changes in the near prescription.

Today the addition can take many forms. These include bifocal or trifocal spectacles, no-line bifocals (such as blended bifocals or PALs), two pairs of glasses, as well as a variety of management strategies involving contact lenses (such as bifocal contacts, overcorrection of contact lenses with reading glasses, simultaneous-vision bifocal contacts, and monovision contacts). The strategy should also be influenced by the patient's needs in terms of the field of vision, psychological issues, and the presence of anisometropia or clinically significant astigmatism. Finally, realizing that the form of the solution to a patient's problem may affect the amount of plus needed, the clinician must be prepared to adjust the near addition after its form has been determined.

References

1. Cline D, Hofstetter HW, Griffin JR. *Dictionary of Visual Science.* 3rd ed. Radnor, Pa: Chilton, 1980:495.

2. Borish IM. *Clinical Refraction.* Chicago: Professional Press, 1975:149–188.

3. Carlson NB, Kurtz D, Heath DA, Hines C. *Clinical Procedures for Ocular Examination.* Norwalk, Conn: Appleton & Lange, 1990:156–160.

4. Carter JH. Determining the nearpoint addition. *N Engl J Optom* 1985;37:4–13.

5. Michaels DD. *Visual Optics and Refraction: A Clinical Approach.* 2nd ed. St. Louis: Mosby, 1980:562–579.

6. Kleinstein RN. Epidemiology of presbyopia. In: Stark L, Obrecht G, eds. *Presbyopia: Recent Research and Reviews from the Third International Symposium.* New York: Professional Press, 1987;12–18.

7. Hofstetter HW. A comparison of Duane's and Donders' tables of the amplitude of accommodation. *Am J Optom Arch Am Acad Optom* 1944;21:345–363.

8. Hofstetter HW. A useful age-amplitude formula. *Penn Optom* 1947;7:5–8.

9. Kaufman PL. Accommodation and presbyopia: neuromuscular and biophysical aspect. In: Hart WM, ed. *Adler's Physiology of the Eye.* St. Louis: Mosby-Year Book, 1992:391–411.

10. Duane A. Studies in monocular and binocular accommodation with their clinical applications. *Am J Ophthalmol* 1922;5:867.

11. Vandepol C, Stark L. Preclinical presbyopic development. In: Obrecht G, Stark LW , eds. *Presbyopia Research: From Molecular Biology to Visual Adaptation.* New York: Plenum, 1991:263–272.

12. Cooper J. Accommodative dysfunction. In: Amos JF, ed. *Diagnosis and Management in Vision Care.* Boston: Butterworth-Heinemann, 1987;431–459.

13. Woo GC, Sivak JG. Factors affecting the reading addition. In: Stark L, Obrecht G, eds. *Presbyopia: Recent Research and Reviews from the Third International Symposium.* New York: Professional Press, 1987:309–313.

14. Testing vision in space part of *Endeavor* mission. *Am Optom Assoc News,* April 15, 1994:1.

15. Milder B, Rubin ML. *The Fine Art of Prescribing Glasses Without Making a Spectacle of Yourself.* Gainesville, Fla: Triad, 1978:101–151.

16. Hanlon SD, Nakabayashi J, Shigezawa G. A critical view of presbyopic add determination. *J Am Optom Assoc* 1987;58:468–472.

17. Sheedy JE, Saladin JJ. Exophoria at near in presbyopia. In: Stark L, Obrecht G, eds. *Presbyopia: Recent Research and Reviews from the Third International Symposium.* New York: Professional Press, 1987:206–210.

18. Hanlon SD. Presbyopia and ocular motor balance. *J Am Optom Assoc* 1984;55:341–343.

19. Kragha IKOK, Hofstetter HW. Bifocal adds and environmental temperature. *Am J Optom Physiol Opt* 1986;63:372–374.

20. Werner DL, Werner WM. Presbyopia and mid-life transition. *Rev Optom* 1979;116(7):43.

21. Ettinger E. *Professional Communications in Eye Care.* Boston: Butterworth-Heinemann, 1994:xiii–xiv.

22. Wilson R. Contemplating presbyopia (editorial). *N Engl J Optom* 1993;45:68.

23. Baron WS. Cyclorotation impacts on toric contact lens fitting and performance. *Optom Vision Sci* 1994;71:350–352.

24. Norman CW. Managing presbyopes with soft contact lenses. *Eye Quest* 1994;Mar/Apr:78–88.

25. Schor C, Erickson P. Ocular dominance, accommodation, and the interocular suppression of blur in monovision. In: Obrech G, Stark LW, eds. *Presbyopia Research: From Molecular Biology to Visual Adaptation.* New York: Plenum, 1991:273–288.

26. Nolan JA, Nolan JJ. Monovision with glasses. *Optom Monthly* 1983;130–133.

27. Erickson P, Schor C. Visual function with presbyopic contact lens correction. *Optom Vision Sci* 1990;67:22–28.

28. Josephson JE, Erickson P, Cattery BE. The monovision controversy. In: Bennett ES, Weissman BA, eds. *Clinical Contact Lens Practice.* Philadelphia: Lippincott, 1993:1–6.

29. Sheedy JE, Harris MG, Gan CM. Does the presbyopic visual system adapt to contact lenses? *Optom Vision Sci* 1993;70:482–486.

30. Back A, Grant T, Hine N. Comparative visual performance of three presbyopic contact lens corrections. *Optom Vision Sci* 1992;69:474–480.

31. Cagnolati W. Acceptance of different multifocal contact lenses depending on the binocular findings. *Optom Vision Sci* 1993;70:315–322.

Case Study Exercises

For each case study, determine the diagnosis and develop a treatment plan. The clinical questions provided with each case may assist you by highlighting important aspects of the case.

Patient C.M.

History: C.M., a 44-year-old trial lawyer, presents with trouble focusing on reading material for the past few months. He is of normal stature and is in excellent health. His job requires a great deal of reading. He has never worn glasses and has no problems with his distance vision.

Clinical Findings		6 m	40 cm
Habitual VA:	OD	20/20	20/30
	OS	20/20	20/30

Amplitude of Accommodation (w/o Rx): 4.00 diopters OD, OS

Keratometry:	OD	43.25/42.87 at 105°
	OS	42.75/43.12 at 75°
Retinoscopy:	OD	+0.25 –0.25 × 100
	OS	plano –0.25 × 45
SRx:	OD	+0.50 DS (20/20)
	OS	+0.25 DS (20/20)

Tentative Add at 40 cm: +1.00 D (20/20)

Phorometry (w/SRx):	6 m	40 cm (w/+1.00 D add)
Phoria	2^ΔEP	2^ΔXP′
BI vergence	8/10/8	10/15/7
BO vergence	10/16/8	12/18/14
NRA/PRA		+1.25/–1.75

Binocular Crossed-Cylinder Add at 40 cm: +1.00 D

Clinical Questions
1. How much add should be prescribed for this patient?
2. What are the lens design options for this add? Which option would likely be the most beneficial for this patient?
3. What are the relevant patient education issues in this case?

Patient C.D.

History: C.D., a 56-year-old travel agent, presents with trouble focusing on reading material even with her reading glasses for the few months before the present visit. Twelve years earlier she obtained her first pair of reading glasses, which she uses over her contact lenses. She is happy with her comfort with her contact lenses, but has noticed that her distance vision is no longer crystal clear through the lenses.

C.D. started wearing contact lenses when she was 22 years of age. She began wearing glasses for distance viewing when she was about 8 years of age. The history indicates that C.D. is following a proper contact lens handling and care regimen. The history is otherwise unremarkable. C.D. is taking no medications.

The habitual spectacle lens prescription (HRx 1) and contact lens prescription (HRx 2) are OD –3.00 DS and OS –3.50 DS. The spectacle lens prescription for near (HRx 3), which is used over the contact lenses is OD +1.25 DS and OS +1.25 DS.

Clinical Findings		6 m (w/HRx2)	40 cm (w/HRx2 + HRx3)
Habitual VA:	OD	20/30	20/25
	OS	20/25	20/30
Amplitude of Accommodation: 2.00 diopters OD, OS			
Keratometry:	OD	41.37/41.87 at 90°	
	OS	41.62/42.12 at 80°	
Retinoscopy:	OD	–3.25 –0.25 × 165	
	OS	–4.00 DS	
SRx:	OD	–3.50 DS (20/20^{+2})	
	OS	–4.00 DS (20/20)	
Tentative Add at 40 cm: +1.75 D (20/20)			

Phorometry (w/SRx):	6 m	40 cm (w/+1.75 D add)
Phoria	ortho	8$^\Delta$XP′
BI vergence	6/8/6	12/16/8
BO vergence	11/15/13	12/22/15
NRA/PRA		+1.00/–0.50
Binocular Crossed-Cylinder Add at 40 cm: +1.75 D		

Clinical Questions
1. How much add should be prescribed for this patient?
2. What are the lens design options for this add?
3. Which option would likely be the most beneficial for this patient?

Patient N.V.

History: N.V., a 64-year-old history teacher, presents with difficulty focusing on reading material for the few months prior even when wearing his reading glasses. He also reports a little blurring of the vision in his left eye at distance, especially at night. N.V. says that he has "funny eyes" and that his eye doctors had always been "very interested in his case." N.V. is in good health and is taking no medications. His history is otherwise unremarkable.

The habitual single vision distance prescription (HRx 1) is OD –1.75 –0.50 × 90 and OS –4.25 –3.25 × 77. The habitual single vision near prescription (HRx 2) is OD +0.25 –0.50 × 90 and OS –2.50 –3.25 × 72.

Clinical Findings		6 m (w/HRx1)	40 cm (w/HRx2)
Habitual VA:	OD	20/20^{-1}	20/30^{-2}
	OS	20/25^{+2}	20/25
Amplitude of Accommodation: 1.00 diopters OD, OS			
Keratometry:	OD	43.12/43.37 at 85°	
	OS	45.25/48.12 at 170°	
Retinoscopy:	OD	–1.50 –0.75 × 100	
	OS	–4.75 –3.50 × 80	
SRx:	OD	–1.50 –0.50 × 90 (20/20^{+1})	
	OS	–4.50 –3.25 × 77 (20/20^{+2})	
Tentative Add at 40 cm: OD +2.25 D and OS +2.00 D (20/20)			

Phorometry (w/SRx):	6 m	40 cm (w/tentative adds)
Phoria	2$^{\Delta}$EP	9$^{\Delta}$XP'
BI vergence	X/9/6	16/19/12
BO vergence	14/16/11	10/12/8
NRA/PRA		+0.50/–0.50

Monocular Crossed-Cylinder Adds at 40 cm: +2.25 D OD, +2.00 D OS

Stereo Acuity at 40 cm (w/SRx and tentative adds): 60 seconds

Ocular Health, Tonometry, and Visual Fields: Normal OU

Clinical Questions
1. Why is the habitual visual acuity of the left eye worse than that of the right eye at distance but better than that of the right eye at near?
2. Are the patient's moderate exophoria and low base-out vergence at near a concern?
3. How much add should be prescribed for this patient? Are unequal adds indicated in this case?
4. What are the lens design options? Which option would likely be most beneficial for the patient?

Patient M.W.

History: M.W., a 50-year-old accountant, presents with trouble focusing on reading material for about the previous 6 months, even with her reading glasses. She has also been disturbed because she feels that she can see better far away with her reading glasses than without them, which is a departure from her first experiences with reading glasses about 10 years ago. M.W. works with fine print in detailed tables and with a computer for at least 6 hours each day. She likes to hold the print at 35 cm and typically views the computer screen from a distance of 70 cm. M.W. is in good health and taking no medication. Her history is otherwise unremarkable. The habitual spectacle prescription for near (HRx) is +1.50 DS OD and OS.

Clinical Findings

Clinical Findings		6 m	40 cm (w/HRx)
Habitual VA:	OD	20/20^{-2}	20/40
	OS	20/20^{-1}	20/30

Amplitude of Accommodation: 4.50 diopters OD, OS

Keratometry:	OD	42.25/42.50 at 90°
	OS	42.50/42.75 at 90°
Retinoscopy:	OD	+1.00 DS
	OS	+0.75 DS
SRx:	OD	+1.25 DS (20/20)
	OS	+1.00 DS (20/20)

Tentative Add at 40 cm: +1.00 D OU (20/20)

Phorometry (w/SRx):	6 m	40 cm (w/+1.00 D add)
Phoria	ortho	8$^\Delta$XP'
BI vergence	7/11/9	9/14/12
BO vergence	13/18/10	22/28/16
NRA/PRA		+1.75/–1.75

Binocular Crossed-Cylinder Add at 40 cm: +1.00 D
Ocular Health, Tonometry, and Visual Fields: Normal OU

Clinical Questions
1. What add should be prescribed for this patient?
2. What are the lens design options for this patient? Which option would likely be the most beneficial for this patient?
3. What is an appropriate treatment plan for this patient?

Appendix: Answers to Clinical Questions

This appendix contains answers to the *Clinical Questions* included with each case study exercise in chapters 2 through 7. It is important to keep in mind that the treatment plans indicated for each of the exercises are samples only, because often more than one plan for a particular patient will adequately resolve the clinical problems.

Chapter 2

Patient J.B.

1. The patient's chief complaint is consistent with the test findings, that is, she has had an increase in myopia.

2. The distance visual acuities with the habitual prescription are consistent with the change of refractive error. The spherical equivalent of the subjective refraction is 0.87 diopter more minus in each eye than the habitual prescription. This is close to the expected amount of uncorrected myopia for the visual acuity observed, as shown in Table 2.1.

3. Because the patient's nearpoint phoria is eso, myopia control may be achieved by the use of a bifocal.

4. An increase in minus power will improve distance visual acuity. Because this will result in nearpoint esophoria, discomfort during nearpoint tasks may result. A plus add may be helpful in reducing nearpoint eyestrain and may serve to slow the rate of progression of myopia. Removal of the glasses would not be a good option for reading, because this would effectively result in a high plus add, and astigmatism would be uncorrected.

5. The subjective refraction (OD –2.75 –1.00 × 90 and OS –2.75 –0.75 × 80) could be prescribed for distance. According to the gradient AC/A ratio, a plus add of +1.00 D would make the near phoria ortho. A flat top 35 mm segment set 2 mm higher than the standard bifocal height would be an effective lens design.

Patient K.C.

1. The symptom of slight distance blur is consistent with a small increase in myopia and with a small improvement in distance visual acuity with the subjective refraction compared with the habitual prescription. The symptoms of ocular discomfort associated with reading can be found in cases of accommodative insufficiency.

2. Having K.C. remove his glasses for near work would not be useful because the effective plus add from the uncorrected myopia would be quite high and because there would be uncorrected anisometropia and uncorrected astigmatism.

3. A small increase in minus would improve distance visual acuity. A plus add would relieve asthenopia associated with accommodative insufficiency.

4. The subjective refraction (OD –5.25 –1.25 × 180 and OS –3.75 –1.75 × 07) could be prescribed for distance. Dynamic retinoscopy suggests a +1.00 D add for near. If confirmed by subjective response with trial framing, the plus add could be provided as multifocal lenses or as a second pair of single vision lenses for reading only.

Patient C.B.

1. The patient's reported lack of vision problems is consistent with the test findings. Distance visual acuity is only slightly better with the subjective refraction than with the habitual prescription, and the accommodation and vergence findings are all within normal limits. There is only a slight change in astigmatism.

2. With an additional –0.25 D added to the subjective refraction to compensate for the 4-meter test distance, the change in spherical equivalent of the subjective refraction compared with the habitual prescription is –0.37 D in each eye.

3. Trial framing would be useful for this patient because she could be shown the effect of an additional –0.37 D on distance vision.

4. A recommendation of new spectacle lenses might be made only if the current lenses are in poor condition, or if the patient feels that her distance vision is much better with the additional –0.37 D. In

that case, the subjective refraction (OD –1.75 –0.25 × 180 and OS –1.50 –0.50 × 173) could be prescribed.

Patient F.E.

1. The patient's chief complaint is consistent with the test finding, because the subjective refraction shows more minus than the habitual prescription.

2. Contact lenses would be an appropriate recommendation for this patient because they would be useful for his sports activities.

3. Less minus is required with contact lenses than with spectacle lenses. The contact lens power can be calculated by use of the effective power formula given in this chapter. For a spectacle correction of –4.75 D and a vertex distance of 14 mm, the calculated contact lens power would be –4.45 D, which would be rounded to –4.50 D.

4. It is advisable that patients have up-to-date spectacle lens corrections even if they have contact lenses. The spectacle lens correction for this patient could be the subjective refraction (OD –4.75 DS and OS –4.75 –0.50 × 180).

Patient A.H.

1. This patient's chief complaint is most likely due to the onset of presbyopia.

2. The subjective refraction shows only a 5° cylinder axis shift from the habitual prescription in each eye. With cylinder powers of 0.25 and 0.50 diopter, this amount of axis change is not enough to cause any difficulty with either distance or near vision. Therefore, in the absence of any other vision problems, a change in lens prescription would not be necessary.

3. A useful prescription would be the subjective refraction for distance (OD –2.50 –0.50 × 170 and OS –2.75 –0.25 × 15) with a +1.00 D add in multifocal form. Although the near phoria with the +1.00 D add is outside the normal range defined by Morgan, the absence of a fixation disparity suggests that the patient will likely not experience fusional vergence difficulty with the add.

Chapter 3

Patient R.B.

1. Given the patient's symptom of tired eyes after 20 minutes of near work, you would expect hyperopia or perhaps an accommodative dysfunction.

2. Considering the patient's uncorrected visual acuity (that is, 20/20 at distance and near) you would expect emmetropia or facultative hyperopia.

3. Javal's rule, that is, $(1.25 \times \text{corneal toricity}) + (0.50 \text{ D against-the-rule})$[3] predicts 0.125 diopter of with-the-rule refractive astigmatism for the right eye and 0.37 diopter against-the-rule for the left eye. However, Javal's rule is not a good predictor with low amounts of corneal toricity. The spherical refractive error found for this patient correlates well with the keratometry readings and with the patient's uncorrected visual acuity at distance and near.

4. The cover test was performed without correction. Because the patient had hyperopia, he would have to accommodate 3.50 diopters during the near cover test (that is, 2.50 diopters for the 40-cm distance at which the test is performed and 1.00 diopter to neutralize the hyperopia). The phoria measured by phorometry was performed with the prescription of +1.00 D OU, thus decreasing the accommodation stimulus to 2.50 diopters and therefore decreasing the esophoria.

5. R.B.'s chief complaint was that his eyes were tired after reading a short period of time. Because he was a student he had substantial near demands. For R.B.'s age (that is, 36 years), Donder's table predicts an amplitude of accommodation of 5.00 diopters. Because R.B. had a near demand of 3.50 diopters without correction, he would need at least 7.00 diopters of accommodation (twice the demand on accommodation) to be comfortable at near. In addition, the near esophoria of 6 prism diopters would add to his discomfort if he had an inadequate supply of negative fusional vergence to compensate for the esophoria. The +1.00 D OU decreases the demand on accommodation, decreases the esophoria, and decreases the demand on negative fusional vergence.

When the +1.00 D OU was demonstrated in a trial frame, R.B. reported that his eyes felt much more comfortable for near work than they did without correction. He also noted that his vision was just as good at distance with the lenses as it was without them. He was advised to wear the lenses for all near work and for distance as he desired. No special lens design is indicated in this case.

Patient T.C.

1. Because the uncorrected visual acuity is more reduced at near than at distance, hyperopia is the expected refractive error.

2. The patient's visual acuity is reduced with correction because of refractive amblyopia. Because the patient had a high amount of hyperopia that had never been corrected, his visual system had never had adequate stimulation and, therefore, had not developed normally.

3. The first treatment for refractive amblyopia is to fully correct the refractive error. In this case, the recommended prescription is +6.50 DS OU. The recommended lens material is polycarbonate. A small eye size for the lens is also suggested to minimize center thickness. The patient should wear the lenses full time. This is often sufficient to increase visual acuity to 20/20. Wearing the lenses only part time will not be as effective in treating the amblyopia.

4. T.C. should be seen for a follow-up examination after 3 months. The clinician should first check the patient's compliance with wearing the lenses. Visual acuity, cover test, stereopsis, and refraction should be evaluated. If the visual acuity has not improved, amblyopia therapy can be started.

5. The prognosis for this patient is excellent if he wears the lenses full time. The parents must be educated about the importance of having the child wear the lenses full time. Full correction of bilateral high refractive error is often sufficient to improve visual acuity to 20/20, but the lenses must be worn full time.

Patient A.L.

1. Because the patient's visual acuity is 20/15 at distance and 20/20 at near, emmetropia or hyperopia is the expected diagnosis.

2. This patient does not need a prescription at this time. She has no vision complaints, her 1.00 diopter of hyperopia can easily be compensated with her accommodation (expected amplitude of accommodation for an 8-year-old is greater than 14.0 diopters, according to Donder's table), and she demonstrated no binocular vision problems without correction.

3. The appropriate treatment plan for this patient would be a re-evaluation in 6 to 12 months to monitor any progression of the hyperopia and identify any vision problems that may develop. A.L.'s parents and teachers should be cautioned about the symptoms and signs of a related vision problem.

Patient R.G.

1. Because the patient's first prescription was dispensed for reading only when he was 42 years of age, R.G. most likely has hyperopia. As a truck driver, he would have to have good vision to pass vision tests on a regular basis to keep his commercial driver's license.

Because the patient is 59 years of age, he would not be expected to have much accommodation, and his hyperopia would be absolute (that is, hyperopia that cannot be neutralized with accommodation). The uncorrected distance visual acuity indicates that R.G. would have about 2.00 diopters of hyperopia in his right eye and about 1.00 diopter of hyperopia in his left eye (that is, approximately one line of Snellen acuity decrease per 0.25 diopter of uncorrected hyperopia).

2. This patient should most certainly be wearing corrective lenses (OD +1.75 –0.25 × 90 and OS +1.00 –0.25 × 90) for driving because his vision is worse than 20/40 in each eye. When the distance subjective refraction findings were trial framed for this patient, he was amazed by how much clearer his distance vision was with the lenses.

3. Progressive addition lenses (+2.25 D add) are recommended for this patient. As a truck driver, he had a variety of distances at which he would need to see clearly, for example, distance for driving, intermediate distances for reading the dashboard, and near for reading maps. R.G. should be told that he did not have to wear the glasses full time; he could wear them for driving, for reading, and any other time that he felt that he needed them. He will likely wear them full time to provide best visual acuity at all distances.

Chapter 4

Patient J.C.

1. The patient holds reading material very close to increase the visual angle of the objects to be seen because the uncorrected visual acuity is so poor.

2. Because J.C.'s uncorrected visual acuities at distance and near are equal, the most likely refractive error is high hyperopia and perhaps astigmatism. High myopia is also a possibility. One would expect that if the myopia were high enough to cause 20/400 acuity at 25 cm, the distance acuity would likely be worse than 20/400.

3. The uncorrected refractive error that would most likely cause the patient's eyes to assume an eso posture at distance and near is hyperopia, because the excessive accommodation used to compensate for the hyperopia results in an overconvergence for the object distances.

4. The amount of astigmatism found during the subjective refraction does correlate with the cylinder found during retinoscopy and the corneal toricity found during keratometry.

5. J.C.'s visual acuity is still reduced after the full plus refraction because of refractive amblyopia. Because his high hyperopia and astigmatism had never been corrected, the patient's visual acuity was always poor and therefore he had never developed the capability for normal acuity.

6. The appropriate treatment plan for the patient would be a full-time prescription. The actual recommended prescription might vary among clinicians, although many practitioners are reluctant to prescribe the full plus found during a cycloplegic refraction, at least as an initial prescription. In this case, a compromise prescription between refraction results with and without cycloplegia (for example, OD +8.00 –4.00 × 130 and OS +9.50 –5.00 × 45) would be suggested to provide the best possible visual acuity and at the same time work toward a full plus prescription. The lenses should be polycarbonate and placed in a sturdy frame.

Adaptation to this unusual prescription is a concern, especially with the oblique cylinder, but any further modification will likely compromise visual acuity. Children tend to be quite adaptable, especially if there is considerable improvement in visual acuity as with this patient. The parents need to be educated about refractive error and amblyopia and informed that the glasses are to be worn full time. A follow-up visit in 1 month is appropriate.

Patient D.A.

1. The patient's history indicates his initial spectacle prescription was dispensed when he was 5 years of age. Knowing that his refractive error was corrected at an early age, and assuming that the high astigmatism in the right eye gradually increased over time, you would not necessarily expect amblyopia to develop. Therefore the normal corrected visual acuity in D.A.'s right eye is not surprising.

2. Because of the nature of the patient's meridional anisometropia, especially in the 40° meridians, one might expect meridional aniseikonia. Considering that D.A.'s aniseikonia is oblique and that he has had a spectacle correction for many years, the absence of this symptom is not unusual.

3. D.A.'s phoria at near of 8^ΔXP' is not a concern because the patient has no symptoms, demonstrates normal stereo acuity, and has a BO vergence at near sufficient to compensate for the exophoria.

4. Because D.A. experiences no problems with his current spectacle prescription and has good visual acuity, no change should be recommended, even though the myopia has increased slightly in each eye and the astigmatism has increased slightly in the right eye with no change of axis. An update of the prescription (for example, –0.25 DS increase OU) might be in order only if the patient desires to change his frame and lenses. Otherwise a re-examination would be indicated in 12 to 18 months.

Patient R.N.

1. The patient's symptoms do suggest a prescription change. The nature of the change is difficult to predict from the symptoms alone.

Considering R.N.'s age, either an increase in hyperopia or astigmatism would cause blurred vision at distance and near.

2.   Esophoria alone does not necessarily correlate with a prescription change unless there in an increase in the phoria from the previous examination. If, for example, the patient experienced exophoria at distance when the habitual lenses were prescribed, esophoria would then suggest that the patient may be accommodating at distance to compensate for some uncorrected hyperopia. The accommodation would then stimulate accommodative convergence.

3.   A change of prescription for high astigmatism may cause some adaptive symptoms regardless of the amount of change. This is especially true if the axis is changed. In this case, the axis at 40 cm changed by 2° from habitual in the left eye and by 1° in the right eye. The cylinder power increased by 0.50 diopter and the sphere power by 0.75 diopter in each eye. The trial frame prescription (OD +1.50 –3.50 × 70 and OS +2.50 –5.00 × 110) provides the spherical equivalent of the subjective at 40 cm by reducing the sphere by 0.25 diopter and the cylinder by 0.50 diopter in each eye and maintains the habitual cylinder axes. The slight increase in plus power would account for the decreased acuity at distance and near with the habitual prescription for a 36-year-old patient.

4.   The appropriate treatment plan would be to dispense a modified prescription that would provide good visual acuity and at the same time minimize adaptive distortion. The modified prescription indicated above provides 20/20 acuity and minimizes spatial distortions. The lens design should include a small eye-size frame with a short vertex distance.

Patient E.P.

1.   The patient's chief complaint is quite consistent with his habitual visual acuities. He reports blurred vision and fatigue at near and is in fact demonstrating reduced acuity at near and distance as well. He does not, however, report blur at distance. An increase in hyperopia by 0.50 diopter OU and slight axis change of the left eye would certainly account for the change of visual acuities and the difference between the right and left eye.

2.   It is not surprising that this patient has no symptoms of spatial distortion considering the high cylinder correction; he has worn such a correction for many years and has adapted well. Apparently when he was first prescribed a correction for astigmatism at age 7, he did experience adaptation symptoms.

3.   The change in the cylinder axes when the subjective refraction is performed at 40 cm as compared with refraction at 6 m is due to the cyclorotation (torsion) of the eyes during convergence. With low cylinders, any axis change may not be apparent to the patient because it will have little effect on acuity, whereas a high cylinder axis change will have a greater effect. This shifting of axis may be clinically significant for a particular patient and therefore must be considered in the prescription. In this case, the shift was not considered clinically significant.

4. A 2° axis change for the left eye with such a high cylinder will likely have a noticeable effect on acuity and may produce some spatial distortion. The change is indicated because the habitual acuity at distance and near of the left eye is slightly worse than that of the right eye. In this case the patient would likely adapt easily to the axis change if it improved visual acuity and caused only a minimal amount of distortion.

5. An appropriate treatment plan for E.P. would include a change of his bifocal prescription to fully correct his hyperopia and replace the scratched lenses, both of which would improve visual acuity at distance and near. No change of add is necessary because adding +0.50 D at distance will also add it at near. The recommended prescription is OD +4.75 −6.50 × 03 and OS +5.75 −8.00 × 177 with a +2.25 D add OU. All lens features (for example, lens material, base curve) should be duplicated. Although a change of the lens material to high index would make the lenses lighter and thinner, it can also create distortion, resulting in symptoms.

A single vision reading prescription (OD +7.00 −6.50 × 03 and OS +8.00 −8.00 × 177) with the optical centers set 2 mm below the geometric centers of the lenses also is recommended to minimize prismatic effect when the patient looks down to read.

Chapter 5

Patient L.L.

1. The lens prescription of choice for this patient is the subjective refraction data (OD −0.75 −0.25 × 180 and OS −3.00 −0.25 × 10), because this prescription provides the best acuity for each eye and balances accommodation. Any modification of the prescription to reduce the difference between the two eyes would only result in a loss of acuity. There will, of course, be an adaptation to this prescription, including possible spatial distortion, and the patient should be so advised.

2. L.L. is expected to demonstrate normal binocular vision with the prescription. His stereo acuity and phorometry data indicate normal binocular function. However, a 2.25-diopter anisometropia may cause aniseikonia, which could interfere with binocularity. In addition, when L.L. looks below the optical centers of the lenses to read, a vertical imbalance will result.

It is often difficult to predict problems for a first-time lens wearer. Each patient should be informed about the symptoms and signs of binocular vision problems that may occur. If the symptoms persist, then a re-evaluation should be made and corrective measures implemented if indicated.

3. First-time wearers of an anisometropic prescription should receive closer follow-up attention than other patients because of the potential adaptation problems. In this case a re-examination should be conducted 1 month after the lenses are dispensed to evaluate L.L.'s progress.

Patient D.T.

1. A treatment plan for D.T. would include single vision lenses with a modified prescription using lens powers between the cycloplegic and noncycloplegic refraction data. In this case, the following would be recommended: OD +5.00 –0.50 × 80 and OS +1.00 DS. This prescription is equal to the noncycloplegic retinoscopic findings and is 1.25 diopters less plus than the cycloplegic retinoscopic findings. The 0.50 diopter cylinder OD is consistent with findings from both retinoscopies. The amount of plus sphere might be increased in the future as the patient adapts to the prescription. A full plus prescription that provides best visual acuity is a desired goal for patients with eso deviations to relax as much accommodation as possible and thereby reduce the deviation.

2. Aniseikonia is most certainly a concern for this patient. However, because best visual acuity is quite poor in the right eye, the patient may never perceive the effects of aniseikonia. However as a precaution, compensation for a shape magnification difference between the lenses may be minimized by either flattening the base curve of the right lens by approximately 4.00 diopters relative to a standard curve or by using a high-index aspheric lens design.

3. Because the patient has deep amblyopia in the right eye due to deprivation of the clear image and ultimately esotropia, vision therapy must be considered in conjunction with the lenses. Although normal binocularity may have a poor prognosis, such therapy may yield some improvement of function.

Patient A.T.

1. A.T.'s feeling of nausea during trial framing with the subjective refraction data was most likely due to the power change of the lenses from her habitual prescription and the varying prismatic effects induced while gazing through different portions of the lenses.

2. The patient's sensation of her eyes "pulling apart" when she drops her eyes to read likely results from an induced vertical prismatic imbalance when she views below the optical centers of the lenses. For example, because the power in the vertical meridian of the right and left eye through the segments is +2.00 D and –1.25 D respectively, a prismatic difference of 3.25^Δ (that is, 2^Δ base up OD and 1.25^Δ base down OS) is produced when the patient looks 10 mm below the optical centers. When she looks through the optical centers, no prismatic difference is present.

3. Additional assessment of the integrity of binocular vision at near in particular would be indicated for this patient, especially if symptoms persist. This assessment should include testing of fusion and aniseikonia with the new prescription.

4. A.T. would benefit from a new prescription for distance and near (OD –0.25 –0.25 × 180 and OS –2.50 –1.25 × 180 with a +2.50 D add OU) to provide best visual acuity. A single vision prescription for reading with the optical centers of the lenses set below the geometric center of the lenses to match the pupil positions when the patient is reading, would be beneficial to minimize vertical prism effects.

The patient should be advised about the nature and origin of her prescription changes, her prescription options, and the likely adaptation period for the new prescription. In this case, A.T. opted for two single vision prescriptions, that is, one for distance only and another for near only, because she was dissatisfied with bifocal lenses.

Patient F.F.

1. Unilateral phoria or asymmetric phoria might occur with uncorrected hyperopia and anisometropia because of an unequal accommodation stimulus during distance viewing. When F.F. is wearing his habitual prescription, his right eye accommodates about 2.00 diopters and the left eye about 0.75 diopter for clear vision at distance. During an alternating cover test, the eye that is covered is forced to converge as a result of accommodation of the fellow eye. If the patient normally exhibited orthophoria at distance, he would now exhibit esophoria of the left eye because of the excessive accommodation of the right eye.

2. The likely cause of the patient's symptom of occasional blur when reading with the habitual prescription is uncorrected hyperopia and anisometropia. F.F. is accommodating an additional 0.75 diopter to 1.75 diopters to provide clearest vision. Fatigue of accommodation would compromise his ability to maintain a clear image, especially under stress.

3. A full plus prescription (that is, cycloplegic retinoscopy data) would not be desirable because cycloplegia eliminates all accommodation. Without cycloplegia, a full plus prescription would likely over-plus the patient's distance vision. Therefore, a modified prescription is usually recommended.

A rule-of-thumb often used to modify plus power is to deduct 1.00 diopter to 1.25 diopters from the cycloplegic sphere to determine the maximum plus to prescribe. In this case the recommended prescription is OD +5.25 –0.50 × 180 and OS +2.00 DS, that is, 1.00 diopter more plus for the right eye and no change for the left eye as compared to the noncycloplegic refraction.

The spectacle lenses should be designed to minimize shape magnification differences by flattening the base curve of the OD lens by approximately 3.00 diopters. This will also serve to improve cosmesis of the lenses. F.F. should be advised of the need for the prescription change and the benefits it will provide for his binocular vision.

Chapter 6

Patient J.R.

1. The patient's uncorrected distance visual acuities are slightly better than one would predict from the habitual prescription. A refractive error of about 1.00 diopter of myopia would likely result in an uncorrected visual acuity of no better than 20/30. Because J.R.'s uncorrected acuity is 20/25, his prescription is probably overminused by at least 0.25 diopter. Even though the prescription is overminused, J.R.'s good amplitude of accommodation can easily compensate for the stimulus to accommodation at distance.

2. Even though J.R.'s prescription is overminused by 0.50 diopter in the right eye and about 0.25 diopter in the left eye, he has no symptoms with the prescription. Often for these patients, a little extra minus at distance is beneficial at very far distances, especially at night. No improvement in acuity is achieved with the refraction findings. Therefore, a prescription change may be indicated only if the patient desires a new frame and lenses, as did this patient. Otherwise no change should be recommended.

3. Because the patient does not wear the prescription for near-point activities and has no symptoms, there is really no indication to recommend otherwise. The patient should continue to remove the glasses for near viewing if he desires. His binocular function at near seems quite normal with or without the prescription.

4. No change of prescription would be recommended for J.R. unless a new frame and lenses were desired. If so, the subjective refraction data could be prescribed if accepted at trial framing. Often in these cases, however, maintaining a little extra minus is preferred by the patient, that is, OD –0.75 –0.25 × 180 and OS –0.75 DS. This prescription would maintain the same refraction balance found during the subjective refraction and would decrease the minus by 0.25 diopter in the right eye and by 0.12 diopter in the left eye.

Patient D.F.

    1. The patient's symptoms alone suggest a variety of causes, such as hyperopia, astigmatism, and accommodation or vergence dysfunction. Because the patient's accommodation and vergence findings are normal for her age, the most likely cause of the symptom of asthenopic headache is low compound hyperopia, especially with oblique principal meridians of the eye. The frequency of the headaches, time of day, and association with a vision task helps the clinician confirm this diagnosis, especially in the absence of other clinically significant findings.

    2. The patient's uncorrected visual acuity is 20/20 with only a very slight improvement with correction (that is, two letters of the 20/15 line OU). The patient therefore may have difficulty appreciating the difference with correction but may feel the quality of the acuity letters improves. She would, however, be expected to notice an improvement in vision comfort when using the lenses over an extended period of time. The use of a trial frame and lenses with a reading task would likely demonstrate this difference.

    3. The patient demonstrates normal phorias and vergences at distance and near except for a low BO vergence at near. Her near point of convergence is also normal. With correction, the near phoria of 4^{Δ}XP′ is adequately compensated with the BO vergence as indicated by the blur point of 12 prism diopters. Even though the blur point is lower than expected, the patient would not necessarily experience any vergence dysfunction. However, if symptoms persist after the ametropia is corrected, this may be an avenue to explore.

    4. The most appropriate treatment plan for this patient would be to correct the low ametropia (OD +0.50 –0.25 × 120 and OS +0.50 –0.25 × 40) using a conventional lens design. The patient should be instructed to use the lenses for all near work and at distance if desired.

Patient R.C.

    1. Considering the patient's age and her uncorrected hyperopia, it is likely that her symptom of blurred vision at near is a result of uncorrected hyperopia alone, because she demonstrates normal visual acuity at near with the distance correction, which therefore precludes a diagnosis of early presbyopia. The correction of the hyperopia provides slight improvement in visual acuity at distance but substantial improvement at near.

2. R.C. is on the threshold of presbyopia that would not be diagnosed as such at this point. The patient is still able to achieve normal visual acuity at near without an add over her distance correction, and she has an amplitude of accommodation equal to 5.00 diopters. Her age alone is not a good indicator of presbyopia, although one does expect beginning symptoms and signs around this age.

3. Corrective lenses are definitely indicated for this patient because she experiences blurred vision at near due to uncorrected compound hyperopia. Because the distance correction only (OD +0.75 –0.25 × 180 and OS +0.75 –0.25 × 175) is indicated to provide normal visual acuity at distance and near, the patient could use the prescription for all distances as she desired. Her priority would be near work, but she would also benefit from using the prescription at distance.

If the patient prefers to use the lenses for near only, the low cylinder correction would probably have little effect on acuity or comfort and therefore could be left out of the prescription. Prescribing the cylinder, however, provides the clearest vision possible at distance if the patient decides to use the lenses for distance at a later date.

4. Because there is no indication for a near add for this patient, the appropriate form for the prescription is single vision. Because the prescription is the same for distance and near, the patient would have no difficulty seeing clearly when reading at a desk and then looking up and across a room.

Patient A.Z.

1. The magnitude of A.Z.'s ametropia is reasonably consistent with his uncorrected visual acuities, although it may be slightly worse than expected. Because the myopia is a spherical equivalent of 0.62 diopter in the right eye and 0.50 diopter in the left eye, one would expect uncorrected acuities between 20/25 and 20/30, depending on the patient's ability to interpret blur of the Snellen letters.

2. A prescription to correct the low myopia is certainly justified because of A.Z.'s difficulty in school and his other symptoms. In this case, the full refraction (OD –0.50 –0.25 × 180 and OS –0.50 DS) is required to provide normal acuity at distance.

3. A.Z.'s phoria at distance and near changes from ortho to eso with the subjective refraction findings in place. The distance phoria is low, but the near phoria is moderate. The BI vergence at near should be sufficient to compensate for the induced esophoria. To offset the esophoria at near and avoid secondary symptoms, the glasses should be removed for all near work. The glasses would then be used only in the classroom for seeing the chalkboard and for other distance tasks as the patient desires.

4. Although the prescription would be part time (that is, for distance only), the low cylinder in the right eye should be incorporated to provide the best visual acuity possible for the distance tasks. However, removing the cylinder would probably not have a substantial effect. Either way would likely be acceptable.

Chapter 7

Patient C.M.

1. C.M., having early presbyopia, requires only a very low plus add at near. The tentative add of +1.00 D provides good visual acuity at 40 cm and is consistent with the binocular crossed-cylinder add. However, the NRA and PRA findings are not equal with this add. If one subscribes to the philosophy that an add that equalizes these two findings (+1.50 D and –1.50 D in this case) is desirable, then a +0.75 D add is best. If this add is combined with the patient's distance prescription, then the total plus at near for the right eye and left eye is +1.25 D and +1.00 D, respectively. This total plus seems to correlate quite well with the patient's uncorrected visual acuities at near. A +1.00 D add would probably be excessive.

2. The lens design options for this patient include the following:
   a. Single vision near lens in a full field frame
   b. Single vision near lens in a half eye frame
   c. Multifocal lens

Considering the occupation of the patient, which probably requires both distance and near vision, option b. or c. would be preferable. The patient would likely opt for the former to avoid adaptation to a multifocal lens. If so, the prescription would be OD +1.25 DS and OS +1.00 DS.

3. For a patient with early presbyopia, it is important to discuss changes of vision, especially at near, which will likely occur in time. The option of a multifocal lens should be discussed as a consideration if the distance prescription increases and the need for corrected vision at distance becomes necessary.

Patient C.D.

1. A guideline to follow when determining an add for a patient with presbyopia is to consider the minimum add that provides best visual acuity at the desired reading distance and the maximum range of clear vision at near. In this case, a +2.00 D add provides good acuity at 40 cm, balances the NRA and PRA findings (+0.75 D and –0.75 D), and will provide a range of clear vision from about 28 to 50 cm. A lower add (for example, +1.75 D) would increase the outer limit of the range but would not balance relative accommodation and would likely result in a slight drop in visual acuity. Trial framing of the add is very important to determine patient acceptance.

2. The lens design options for this patient include:
a. Single vision contact lenses for distance with a single vision spectacle prescription to use over the contact lenses for reading
b. Multifocal contact lenses or monovision lenses
c. Single vision or multifocal spectacle lenses

3. Option a. above would be the most beneficial for the patient because she was using this combination of lenses with satisfaction. There would be no reason to change from this option unless the patient desired to do so. The recommended prescription in this case would be OD –3.50 DS and OS –4.00 DS contact lenses for distance combined with single vision +2.00 DS OU for use over the contact lenses when reading. This combination will provide a plus add at near which is 0.25 diopter greater for each eye than the habitual prescription.

Patient N.V.

1. The habitual visual acuity of the left eye is worse than that of the right eye at distance because the patient's habitual single vision distance prescription is underminused by 0.25 diopter OS and overminused by a 0.25 diopter OD. The habitual single vision near prescription is also underminused OS and therefore provides a higher add than the OD. Comparing the difference between the habitual prescription for near and the new refraction data, the patient was habitually wearing a +1.75 D add OD and a +2.25 D add OS.

2. In advanced presbyopia, moderate to high exophoria at near combined with a low BO vergence is not unusual. Surprisingly, relatively few patients with presbyopia with these findings have symptoms related to a convergence insufficiency. In this case, N.V.'s symptoms related to accommodation dysfunction and not to convergence dysfunction.

3. The patient's habitual prescriptions indicate that unequal adds were prescribed by the previous clinician (+2.00 D add OD and +1.75 D add OS). The monocular crossed-cylinder test at 40 cm indicates unequal adds as well. In this case, unequal adds are indicated from both the history and clinical findings. Also, unequal adds were

necessary to provide equal visual acuity at near. Therefore, there is a strong indication that they should be continued. The adds of choice would be +2.25 D OD and +2.00 D OS over the current subjective refraction data (OD –1.50 –0.50 × 90 and OS –4.50 –3.25 × 77), because these adds do balance the NRA and PRA and provide equal acuities at near. Confirmation of patient acceptance should be obtained by use of a trial frame and lenses.

4. The lens design options for this patient include:
   a. Single vision lens for distance and near
   b. Multifocal lens
   c. Contact lenses for distance with spectacle lenses for near
   d. Multifocal contact lenses or monovision lenses

The history did not indicate any patient inconvenience with using two single vision prescriptions rather than multifocal lenses. A good rule-of-thumb is to duplicate the prescription form that has been successful unless the patient desires to make a change. If the patient does want a change, the other options can be considered. In any case, each patient should be informed of these options. The two prescriptions for this patient could be OD –1.50 –0.50 × 90 and OS –4.50 –3.25 × 77 for distance and OD +0.75 –0.50 × 90 and OS –2.50 –3.25 × 72 for near. Note the 5° axis difference for the left eye between the distance and the near prescriptions. This difference existed in the habitual prescriptions and therefore should be maintained because there is usually a shift of the axis of moderate to high cylinder corrections between distance and near viewing. This difference can be confirmed with clinical testing.

Patient M.W.

1. The optimal add for this patient would be one that provides adequate visual acuity at both 35 and 70 cm. Both the tentative add at 40 cm and that found during the binocular crossed-cylinder test indicate an add of +1.00 D. This add also balances the NRA and PRA. Because the patient has an amplitude of 4.50 diopters (which is a little higher than expected for her age), a +1.00 D add should provide good acuity at the required distances. This add represents an increase in her net near prescription of +0.75 D OD and +0.50 D OS. This change is expected, considering the patient's reduced visual acuity at near with the habitual near prescription.

2. Because this patient may benefit from a distance prescription for her hyperopia, the lens design options are as follows:
   a. Single vision lenses for distance and near
   b. Single vision lenses for near only
   c. Multifocal lenses

d. Contact lenses for distance with a single vision lens for near

e. Multifocal contact lenses or monovision lenses

If the patient expresses no interest in contact lenses, then option a., b., or c. should be considered. Because M.W.'s habitual prescription was a single vision lens for near, and considering that she appreciated the improved vision at distance with correction, option a. or c. would likely be the most beneficial for this patient.

3. A recommended prescription would be OD +1.00 DS and +0.75 DS OS with a +1.25 D add OU. The total plus at distance was reduced by 0.25 diopter to ensure best possible visual acuity at distances greater than 6 meters. This is an important consideration, especially for a patient with hyperopia who has reasonably good acuity without a correction. This 0.25 diopter was then added at near so that the total plus at near distances would not be reduced (that is, the add is +1.25 D instead of +1.00 D).

The form of this prescription could be either two single vision prescriptions for distance and near or a multifocal lens. A patient who does not necessarily require a distance prescription full time, as in this case, may opt for single vision lenses to avoid adaptation to multifocal lenses.

Glossary

The following is a list of abbreviations and symbols and the corresponding definitions used in this book.

BI base-in prism

BO base-out prism

D diopter

DS diopter sphere

EDS equivalent diopter sphere or spherical equivalent

EP esophoria at far

EP' esophoria at near

ET esotropia at far

ET' esotropia at near

FT flat top segment

HRx habitual spectacle lens prescription

NPC near point of convergence

NRA negative relative accommodation

OD right eye

OS left eye

OU both eyes

PAL progressive addition lens

PH pinhole aperture

PRA positive relative accommodation

Rx spectacle lens prescription

SRx subjective refraction data

VA visual acuity

XP exophoria at far

XP′ exophoria at near

XT exotropia at far

XT′ exotropia at near

w/ with

w/o without

Δ prism diopter

Index

AC/A (accommodative
    convergence/
    accommodation), 19, 52
Accommodation
    dark focus of, 20
    defined, 147
    distance influence factors,
        151–152
    customary near tasks,
        151–152
    patient stature, 151
    patient's ametropia and lens
        effectivity, 152
    vocational and avocational
        considerations, 152
    physiologic stimulus to, 153–154
Accommodative esotropia, 55
Accommodative excess, 20
Accommodative spasm, 20
Acuity
    best visual, 102
    reduced distance visual, 15
    visual, 4–7
Age related to myopia, 16
Amblyopia
    meridional, 75
    refractive, 75
    refractive or strabismic
        amblyopia, 52

American Optical Office-
        Model space eikonometer,
        104
Ametropia
    and asthenopia, 2
    and blurred vision, 2
    clinical analysis, 7–9
    clinical analysis of, 1–11
    clinical questions, 8–9
    clinical rule-of-thumb, 4–5
    diagnosis, 8
    historical notes, 1
    low, 123–143
    management of, 1–11
    management with spectacle
        lenses, 9–10
    principles of patient care, 10
    rules-of-thumb, 6
    symptoms and signs, 2–3
    treatment plan, 8
    uncorrected, 4–7
    and viewing distance, 3
Aniseikonia
    clinical management of, 104
    defined, 102–103
    history, 104
    managing, 104
    predicting the amount of,
        105

Anisometropia, 99–121
  clinical management of, 102
  hyperopic, 101
  myopic, 101
  prescription guidelines,
      101–106
    amblyopia and strabismus,
        102–103
    aniseikonia, 103–105
    binocular vision, 105–106
    refractive error and best visual
        acuity, 102
  refractive or axial, 104
  symptoms and signs of, 101
Anisometropic hyperopia, 52
Anisophoria, optical, 106
Antimetropia, 101
Asthenopia
  causes of, 2–3
  defined, 2
  headaches and, 3
  onset of symptoms, 3
  symptoms, 50, 126
Astigmatism, 73–98
  bilateral, 78–79
  full prescription versus a partial
      prescription, 76
  irregular, 77
  mixed, 6
  myopic, 77
  prescription guidelines,
      75–82
    accommodation and
        vergence, 78–79
    age of the patient, 75
    first-time, 78
    habitual lens wear, 78
    meridional aniseikonia,
        79
    severity, 77
    special lens design
        considerations, 81
    spectacle design, 80–81
    vocational and avocational
        considerations, 81–82
  simple myopic, 6
  symptoms and signs of, 75
  types of, 77
  uncorrected, 5, 126

Bifocal contact lenses, window, 160
Bifocal lenses, 157
Bilateral astigmatism, 78–79
Blur, intermediate, 155
Blurred vision, 2, 125

Central (foveal) suppression, 102
Childhood myopia, 17
Clinical analysis defined, 7
Clinical rule-of-thumb (ametropia),
    4–5
Coatings, antireflection, 21
Compound myopia defined, 6
Congenital myopia, 16
Contact lenses; see also Hyperopia;
    Presbyopia
  rigid gas-permeable, 24, 26
  simultaneous vision bifocal, 161
  window bifocal, 160
Convergence, fusional, 128
Culture, youth, 157
Customary near working distance,
    151
Cycloplegic refraction, 20
Cycloplegic refractions, 51, 54
Cylinder axis
  measuring change in, 79
  nearpoint, 76–77

Dark focus of accommodation, 20
Dictionary of Visual Science, 2, 147
Distometer defined, 23
Distortions, spatial, 76, 81
Double vision, 2

EDS (equivalent diopter sphere)
    examples, 5–6
Emmetropia, 20, 50
Esophoria, 19
  nearpoint, 24
Esotropia, accommodative, 55
Ethnicity and myopia, 16
Excess, accommodative, 20
Exotropia, 19
Eyestrain, patients with symptoms
    of, 126

Facultative hyperopia, 50
Fear, ocular, 126
Fusional convergence, 128

Glasses, multiple pairs of 160; *see
    also* Lenses; Spectacle lenses

Hyperopia, 45–71
    amplitude of accommodation,
        50
    anisometropic, 52
    changes little throughout life,
        49
    defined, 49
    facultative, 50
    latent, 51
    low to moderate, 153
    partial hyperopic prescriptions,
        51
    patients who need a partial
        correction, 50–51
    prescription guidelines, 50–56
        accommodation and vergence,
            51–52
        adult hyperopia, 50–51
        contact lenses, 55–56
        first-time and habitual lens
            wearers, 53
        pediatric hyperopia, 53–55
        severity, 52–53
        spectacle lens and frame
            design, 55
    shift toward, 16
    symptoms and signs of, 4–50
Hyperopic anisometropia, 101

Intermediate blur, 155
Iseikonic lens designs, 81

JCC (Jackson crossed-cylinder)
    power refinement, 78

Keratometry, 25
Knapp's law, 104, 158

Latent hyperopia, 51
Lenses; *see also* Spectacle lenses;
    Glasses
    high minus, 22
    iseikonic, 81, 105
    low-power spectacle, 128
    multifocal, 159
    polycarbonate, 22
    progressive addition, 159
    spectacle, 9–10
Lenses, spectacle design, 21–23
    antireflection coating, 22
    antireflection coatings, 21
    appearance of rings, 22
    edging procedures, 21–22
    high minus lenses, 22
    rolling and polishing, 22
    weight of, 22
Low ametropias, 123–143
    case history of a patient with, 126
    diagnosis of, 125–126
    and patient anxiety, 126
    personality types related to, 126
    prescription, 126–129
    prescription guidelines, 126–129
        accommodation and vergence,
            128
        benefits of corrective lenses,
            127–128
        management strategy, 127
        spectacle design, 128–129
        symptoms affect patients of all
            ages, 126–127
        treatment plan, 128
    symptoms and signs of, 124–126
Low myopia, 126

Meridional amblyopia, 75
Mixed astigmatism defined, 6
Multifocal lenses, 159
Myopia, 13–43
    accommodation and
        convergence requirements,
        19
    accommodative infacility, 15
    childhood, 17
    classification and prevalence of,
        15–16

Myopia (*continued*):
  compound, 6
  congenital, 16
  control of, 23–26
  correction for, 21–23
  decrease in visual acuity, 4
  distance blur (symptom), 14
  and ethnicity, 16
  lens reflections, 21
  low, 126
  measurement of, 20–21
  night, 20
  and presbyopia, 18
  prescription guidelines, 17–26
    accommodation and vergence,
      19–20
    adaptation to lenses, 17
    change of refractive error, 17
    patients who can read without
      glasses, 19–20
    uncorrected astigmatism, 17
  progression of, 16–17
  refractive changes with age,
    16–17
  refractive error changes, 21
  relation to age, 16
  sign of, 15
  spectacle lens design, 21
  spectacle-corrected, 152–153
  symptoms and signs of, 14–15
  and years of education, 16
Myopia control
  defined, 23
  use of bifocal lenses, 23–24
Myopic anisometropia, 101
Myopic astigmatism, 6, 77

Near working distance, customary,
  151
Nearpoint cylinder axis, 76–77
Night myopia, 20
Noncycloplegic refraction, 51

Ocular fear, 126
Optical anisophoria, 106
Overrefractions (contact lenses), 23

PALs (progressive addition lenses),
  82, 155, 157, 159
Patient care, management of
  ametropia, 10
Polycarbonate lenses, 22
Presbyopia, 76, 145–179
  accommodation demand,
    assessing the need, 150–154
  contact lens treatment options
    for, 160–162
    bifocal contact lenses
      (alternating vision), 160
    contact lenses for distance, 162
    monovision, 161–162
    overcorrection for contact
      lenses, 160–161
    simultaneous vision bifocal
      contact lenses, 161
  defining, 147–148
  onset of, 147–148
  patients with, 53
  prescription guidelines, 149–158
    amplitude of accommodation,
      149–150
    anisometropia, 158
    astigmatism, 158
    effects of distance prescription
      changes, 156
    field of vision, 156–157
    intermediate blur, 155
    net near prescription, 156
    plus adds and exo deviation,
      155–156
    psychological issues, 157–158
    range of clear vision, 154–155
    visual acuity, 154–155
    what is a "normal" add?, 156
  spectacle lens treatment options
    for, 158–160
    multifocal lenses, 158–159
    multiple pairs of glasses, 160
    no-line multifocal lenses, 159
  symptoms and signs of, 148–149
  and use of trifocals, 159
Prescription, accuracy of the lens,
  22
Progressive addition lenses, 159
Pseudomyopia, diagnosis of, 20

Ratio, accommodative convergence/accommodation (AC/A), 52
Refractions
    cycloplegic, 20, 51, 54
    noncycloplegic, 51
    objective and subjective data, 125
    subjective, 20–21
Refractive amblyopia, 53–54, 75
Refractive balance, improper, 102
Refractive errors present at birth, 16
Refractive or strabismic amblyopia, 52
Rules-of-thumb
    ametropia, 4–5
    aniseikonic symptoms, 105

Scientific method defined, 7
Simple myopic astigmatism defined, 6
Spasm, accommodative, 20

Spatial distortions, 76, 81
Spectacle lenses; see also Lenses; Glasses
    and ametropia, 9–10
    low-power, 128
Spectacle-corrected myopia, 152–153
Subjective refraction, 20–21

Uncorrected low astigmatism, 126
Underconvergence, 128

VDTs (video display terminals) and vision related symptoms, 125
Vertex distance defined, 22–23
Vision
    blurred, 2, 125
    double, 2
    symptoms related to VDTs, 125
Visual acuity, 4–7
    decrease in, 4
    reduced distance, 15